Caregiving
Both Ways

Caregiving Both Ways

A Guide to Balancing It All While
Caring for a Loved One
with Dementia

Molly Wisniewski

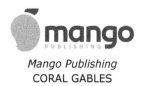

Mango Publishing
CORAL GABLES

Published by Mango Publishing Group, a division of Mango Media Inc.
Cover Design: Roberto Núñez
Cover Photo/illustration: TierneyMJ (Shutterstock)
Layout & Design: Jayoung Hong
For permission requests, please contact the publisher at:

Mango Publishing Group

2850 S Douglas Road, 2nd Floor

Coral Gables, FL 33134 USA

info@mango.bz

For special orders, quantity sales, course adoptions and corporate sales, please email the publisher at sales@mango.bz. For trade and wholesale sales, please contact Ingram Publisher Services at customer.service@ingramcontent.com or +1.800.509.4887.

Caregiving Both Ways: A Guide to Balancing It All While Caring for a Loved One with Dementia

Library of Congress Cataloging-in-Publication number: 2019941763

ISBN: (print) 978-1-63353-984-6, (ebook) 978-1-63353-985-3

BISAC category code: MEDICAL / Caregiving

Printed in the United States of America

To my husband, Kevin: You are my favorite person, and I appreciate your continued enthusiasm and support!

Table of Contents

Chapter Ten

Foreword

By Carol Bradley Bursack, Minding Our Elders

Every caregiver has a unique story to tell, most often one of jumbled emotions that cycle through times of joy, despair, grief, and gratitude. My decades-long journey was a juggling act that was, while also unique to my circumstances, no different when it came to emotions.

For me, caregiving began with my neighbor, Joe, who had lived with Meniere's disease since his thirties and, as a result, was completely deaf. When Joe was in his eighties, his wife died. That left him alone except for some older friends from his working years and his only adult child, who lived across the country. We hadn't socialized before, other than giving a wave and saying "hi," because Joe seemed busy with his life and I had a young family. But now? How could a neighbor not offer to help?

Back then, my children were young. Over time, we grew to love Joe, but, as I crossed our yards that first day to see if I could do anything to comfort this seemingly vulnerable older man, I had no way of knowing that I was entering into an unspoken contract to be Joe's caregiver for the next five years. Still, I don't see that I could have done things differently, and I wouldn't have wanted to miss those years, even if I'd had the chance to do it over.

During my "Joe years," as I call them, my aunt and uncle, who had no children, moved from the Washington, DC, area to be near my family. They even moved into the same apartment complex as my parents. We were all close, and my siblings and I were my aunt and uncle's substitute kids, so this was the natural progression of life.

For a few years, life was good for all of my family elders. They even took a couple of cruises together. Meanwhile, I was busy with young children and Joe's needs. We visited my parents, aunt and uncle, and in-laws regularly and did an occasional favor, as any adult child would do, but I wasn't needed then as a caregiver.

Then, shortly after Joe's death, my uncle had his first stroke, which seemed to trigger a chain reaction when it came to my family's elder health. My trips to emergency rooms, doctors' offices, and even the occasional hospital room rapidly increased as one by one each elder entered what was, for them, going to be years of poor health. Looking back, I can see that this was the beginning of the end for them all, even though life as such would go on for most of them for more than a decade.

This is what I call the sneak-up effect of caregiving. I handled each crisis as a unique occurrence that I needed to deal with. Yet, with each health emergency, my overall involvement grew. I was deeply involved before I understood that there was no going back, even if I'd chosen to do so. My uncle's strokes introduced us to in-home health care. My mom's less than stellar second hip replacement offered me one of my first experiences of personally providing daily care for an elder. It was, however, my dad's disastrous brain surgery that truly changed all of their lives and made me the caregiver that I would become.

Dad had suffered a brain injury in the service during World War II. Still, after weeks in a coma and much therapy, he went on to lead a successful life in public health. Decades later, the injury came back to haunt him, and fluid began to build up behind the scar tissue in his brain. There were few signs of any cognitive issues when Dad saw the doctor, but still, he rightly recommended surgery to place a shunt in Dad's brain in order to drain what would eventually become increasing amounts of built-up brain fluid into his abdominal cavity. This is a common procedure that's often used for people who have suffered brain injuries, or who develop fluid as they age. It's most often safe and effective. Until it isn't.

Dad's situation, sadly, was one of those times where the surgery, while technically "successful," was a disaster. He came out of that operation with severe dementia, something that he'd live with for the final decade of his life.

Meanwhile, my other elders were beginning to experience health emergencies. My uncle continued having strokes. My aunt collapsed, was hospitalized, was found to be full of cancer and, within weeks, was dead. My father-in-law began to grow frail and suffer small strokes. Eventually, he had one major stroke that hospitalized him, and then kept having strokes until he died.

My mother-in-law, who at the time of her husband's illnesses was having some cognitive issues, grew much worse. Over the course of time, I went to her condo daily and helped with meals, grooming, and other care, and kept her company. Eventually, she moved across the avenue from her condo into the nursing home where, at that time, my dad and uncle lived.

Meanwhile, my mother began falling regularly. At least once a week I would be summoned by an operator managing her emergency alert service. I'd race to Mom's apartment, where I'd just been a couple of hours before, in order to handle the newest emergency, often by calling 911. Additionally, Mom's overall pain worsened, and she began to show dementia symptoms.

After a few years of this routine, she too would join the others in the nursing home.

Some ask why I didn't take one or another of my elders into my home. My answer to this question, which no one should ever ask, is this: I had five elders to care for at one time. Not only didn't I have the type of home to accommodate the needs of that many people, but I was also trying to care for a chronically ill son who was often home from school. When I wasn't with him, I was running from location to location to help my other elders who needed me. No one would have benefited from being shoehorned into my home when there were other choices.

The nursing home that we used, Rosewood on Broadway, was an excellent facility and near all of my elders when they needed it the most. Perhaps even more importantly, it was only two blocks from my home, as well, since I became the chauffeur for those who still lived in their own homes. Since I was still raising children, convenience was paramount. From the beginning, I was well aware that not everyone can find a conveniently located, wonderful facility for their multiple elders, so this stroke of good fortune was something for which I've always been grateful.

Taking into account the six weeks that Joe spent at Rosewood after breaking his hip, I spent a total of fifteen years as a daily visitor at the facility, and the staff became nearly as close as family. To this day, on the rare occasion that I run into one of the nurses or aides while out shopping, tears will flow on both sides as memories are recalled.

One by one, over the course of those fifteen years, my elders grew extremely ill and, one by one, they left us to go to a better place. I still feel them all with me, only now they are strong, free, and once again happy.

During all of those years, there was little help for caregivers. What we did was simply expected of women, and we received as much respect as a piece of old furniture. So, from just becoming a caregiver to avoiding caregiver burnout—a completely foreign concept to me—to dementia care, which the medical community had all wrong at the time, to navigating in-home care, nursing homes, and legal issues, I truly was on my own.

Now, fortunately, there are resources galore. Books, such as the one that you are about to read, are invaluable. There are online support groups, disease-specific websites, and caregiver forums. Take advantage of them all for information, as well as companionship, as you travel down your own caregiving path.

I want to leave you with a few suggestions gleaned from my time in the trenches:

- Educate yourself about your older adult or spouse's specific condition. Disease-specific sites, as suggested above, are a godsend.

- Join a caregiver support group in person if you can, online for certain. Ideally, both. You can't have too much support.

- Do your personal best, whether that means caring for your vulnerable friend, relative, or loved one in their home, taking them into yours, or using the services of a care facility. One caregiver's best may be to hire people to provide all hands-on care while they coordinate things from the office, or even from a distance. Another caregiver's best may be providing around-the-clock care in their own home. Each situation is unique.

- Don't criticize other caregivers and don't accept criticism from them. Most of us do what we can with what circumstances allow.

- There's no such thing as a perfect caregiver, so do not let guilt eat at you. Most caregiver guilt is unearned. Let it go. If you can improve, find out how. If it's too late to improve, accept that you did your best with what you had at the time. Either way, let go. Let go. Let go. Your feeling guilty won't help anyone.

- Give yourself credit for putting in your time doing what needed to be done. Take advantage of the abundance of information now available. Pace yourself the best you can so you can withstand what is likely to become a marathon event. Do the best you can with what you have, and you'll do fine.

Introduction

My name is Molly Wisniewski, and I've worked with older adults for over ten years. I was fortunate to begin my career with a mentor who was dedicated to the teaching of resident rights and a strong advocate for quality of life and quality of care for our seniors living in nursing homes. Her energy and passion ignited my desire to continue her work and share a more positive side of the aging experience.

Over the years, I've watched as family members struggled with challenging behaviors associated with various forms of dementia or Alzheimer's disease. The loss of memory, language, and even direction is hard to witness and understand. For family caregivers, there is a lifetime of memories which have seemingly disappeared from your loved one's mind.

My project, the Upside to Aging, started as a way to address this very concern. The focus is to offer resources and education to family members who are hurt and confused by their loved one's behavior and who struggle with the shift of power that abruptly occurs as they assume the caregiver role. Many of the entries found on my website have been expanded in this book to offer key examples of how to interact and engage your loved one living with dementia.

Caregivers cannot provide proper care without understanding the behaviors of these individuals. My experience working with older adults taught me several things; however, what I will dedicate this book to is the understanding and awareness that older adults with various forms of dementia are not behaving in a certain way because of their diagnosis, but instead, they are communicating with us in a new way. We just need to learn the language.

Through this lens, we can gain awareness, understanding, and even empathy toward their needs and allow both family and professional caregivers to get to know these individuals in a new way during this phase of life. My professional and educational background is in caregiving and aging, not medicine, and this is my approach to the diagnosis here. I have spent countless hours getting to know individuals with dementia, have identified patterns in behavior and the intonation of voice, and have established relationships that I still hold dear today.

Dementia is a group of symptoms that have an impact on the cognitive health of the person diagnosed, and there are several stages a person will go through and various levels of capability throughout the progression of their life post-diagnosis. In this book, I will focus on care techniques and interventions for individuals who need assistance with activities of daily living and who are in later stages of the disease process.

To provide skilled care to someone living with dementia is a unique caregiving experience, and there are established tools out there to make the experience as comfortable for both parties as possible. Unfortunately, there isn't a training period for family caregivers and, to best be able to provide care to someone living with later-stage dementia, the caregiver must understand how the individual has re-learned to communicate. Too often individuals living with dementia are passed over because there is a general belief that these people can no longer comprehend or communicate, but this is far from the truth. Your loved one is very much still alive inside and is waiting for you to engage them in a way that they can respond to and understand.

In the first part of this book, I explore the very nature of a caregiver and what impact caregiving for a loved one has on the relationship with the care recipient. Chapter One will go over the variety of settings in which caregivers work and live, and acknowledge the need for our communities to support this growing subset of our population. Chapter Two focuses on you, the caregiver. You are in a demanding role that can quickly burn you out if you don't take time for yourself. Each section will provide you with new tools to help you incorporate self-care into your routine. Chapter Three hones in on the language of dementia. So much of the caregiver's frustrations stem from misunderstanding their loved one's needs and preferences. Paying attention to subtleties in speech patterns and identifying dementia triggers will help you better understand what it is your loved one is trying to tell you. Chapter Four offers a series of interventions that calm and redirect an individual living with dementia. Chapter Five focuses on the importance of activities, and how engaging your loved one in certain recreational pursuits can help you provide care as a family caregiver.

The second part of this book focuses on the importance of caregiving conversations in the relationship between caregivers and care recipients. To that end, Chapter Six acknowledges the difficulties in care and offers mindful caregiving techniques to support you in your approach. Then Chapter Seven sets the foundation for your care conversation with your loved one and provides context and questions that will help you clearly outline their wishes and preferences. Next, Chapter Eight goes over the growing number of senior living options available on the market and seeks to debunk the idea that nursing homes are the only option for your loved one in need of care. Chapter Nine discusses what you should look for when searching for a care home for your loved one, acknowledges the guilt that many caregivers have for moving their loved one into a nursing home, and offers concrete examples of how you can remain an active participant in their care. Chapter Ten recognizes the continued role of the caregiver once their loved one has passed away and offers ways to memorialize the times spent together throughout the caregiving journey.

As an activity professional, I am continuously humbled by the joy, kindness, and compassion these individuals have in their hearts, and their willingness to share this love with all those they meet. I hope that you, too, can find these relationships with the older adults living with dementia or Alzheimer's disease in your life.

Part One

How to Ease Care through Activity Engagement

Chapter One

The Unexpected Family Caregiver

The caregiver is often considered a hero. We acknowledge how difficult it is to care for someone else, and, while there are programs and support systems in place to advocate for the family caregiver, the bulk of the work is left to you to handle. The joyful moments spent with someone living with dementia or Alzheimer's are great, and I've had the honor of developing relationships with many individuals living with this disease. These moments, however, are formed outside the daily care routine. I've witnessed firsthand the struggles between caregivers and care recipients as they navigate the most delicate aspects of care. These intimate moments of caregiving hold a vulnerable part of the human experience, and one that should never be taken lightly.

The start of a caregiving journey will be different for everyone because the role of a caregiver can be brought on by an acute illness, or maybe you've assisted in a family member's care for years without realizing: a trip to the doctor's office, scheduling appointments, or light housekeeping. Often the tasks are easy enough, and for many people, these roles and responsibilities are taken on without much thought. As the family, many assume it is just part of what's required or expected.

Whether it is a spouse, a parent or sibling, grandparent, aunt, an uncle, or whoever raised you, they are older now and need a bit more assistance in their day-to-day activities. The process all seems innocent enough, but, as care demands increase, taking care of your loved one can unexpectedly begin to intrude on your daily routine, job, family, health, and finances. Without a proper plan in place, caregiving becomes a much more complicated process for family members to navigate.

While the word care may be in it, caregiving is practical and medically driven, which leaves very little time for emotional care and relationship building. Continued focus on a person's physical well-being can be both draining and stressful. As we move forward throughout this book, the acknowledgment of feelings of stress, guilt, and even anger is essential. So many caregivers have expressed these sentiments in whispered tones, as if they were wrong or something they should be ashamed of feeling. They are not. These thoughts are healthy and come from being put in a difficult situation. What matters is the way you choose to handle these thoughts.

Due to the sensitive and delicate nature of providing care, it is essential that both parties agree to the care arrangements. The care recipient should express either verbally or in writing what kinds of care measures they agree to, who they want to be providing this care, and an agreement with that person that they are willing and able to take on the role. The caregiver should identify what kinds of care they can provide and understand in what aspects of care they will require additional assistance. Unfortunately, this is hardly ever the case. As mentioned above, family members take on the role unassumingly, and too often without a conversation with the older adult in need. Society tells you to plan for retirement, but the conversation often stops there and neglects to prepare for, or even discuss, a time when you are no longer able to care for yourself.

Longevity is a relatively new concept in our society. Black men who were born in 1950 had a life expectancy of fifty-nine; white men were expected to live to sixty-seven. Today, this is retirement age. Meanwhile, white women who were born in 1950 had a life expectancy of seventy-five; black women were expected to live to sixty-three.[1] Medical advancements and a better understanding and appreciation of nutrition and exercise have resulted in longer and healthier lives for both men and women. We never needed to make plans past retirement because no one expected even to live that long, so now, as we navigate the complexities of an aging population, planning becomes much more relevant and necessary.

To not have these conversations leaves family members to struggle to make the "right" decision for their loved one without knowing what they would want. For instance, AARP (American Association of Retired Persons) and the Centers for Disease Control report that 87 percent of adults over the age of sixty-five have expressed the desire to age in place (to live in one place through every stage of the aging process)[2,3]. However, to make aging in place a sustainable option takes a lot of planning and a lot of money. This, coupled with the less than ideal reputation of nursing homes and other senior care facilities, creates added pressure in deciding whether your loved one should come and live with you. I've had many conversations over the years with people who say "that is just what you do"; however, living with a parent or having the parent come live with you is a significant decision, and there are a lot of factors that should be considered

---

1 Senior Living, https://www.seniorliving.org/history/1900-2000-changes-life-expectancy-united-states/.

2 AARP, *AARP Livable Communities* "Baby Boomer Facts on 50 Livable Communities and Aging in Place," AARP, accessed April 1, 2019, https://www.aarp.org/livable-communities/info-2014/livable-communities-facts-and-figures.html.

3 Centers for Disease Control and Prevention (CDC), *The State of Aging & Health in America 2013* (2013), accessed April 1, 2019, https://www.cdc.gov/aging/pdf/state-aging-health-in-america-2013.pdf

before living together. Not everyone has a good relationship with their parents, but that doesn't mean you won't have to care for them. Don't make the situation worse for yourselves by creating little to no space to step away from the caregiving situation.

The right care setting is out there for all of us; it just takes time and consideration. No doubt, if you have taken on the role of caregiver—no matter your relationship with your loved one— you want the best for them. Sometimes that means you are the primary caregiver, and sometimes it does not. If your loved one hasn't made a decision on how they would like their care handled, or if they assume you are the person for the job without discussing it with you, you have every right to decide for yourself if this is what you want to do. You are not a bad person for saying that the emotional and physical toll of caregiving is just a bit too much for you to take on.

There are a variety of ways you can provide care for your loved one. Getting to know them during this new phase of their life is so important, and, when left to focus primarily on the physical care, this special time together can become muddled with stressful moments. You deserve to look back on this time with joy and love.

Accessing education or resources to learn how to provide care can be difficult. It's not that there is a lack of information on the topic; rather, because caregiving is such a personal experience, it is hard to know where to start. But it is important that you know you are not alone. There are both experts and other family caregivers out there, advocating and educating based on their own experience, and they are more than happy to share what they have learned along the way to help you.

The Caregiver Generation

The role of the caregiver can be found in almost every generation, and, over time, our understanding and recognition of the caregiver's role has been extended beyond the family. Over the past three generations, there has been a dramatic shift in the expectations of who gives care and the extent of the caregiving demands assumed by those individuals providing care. I started work in senior living in 2005 on a skilled nursing unit, and while I didn't know it at the time, the demographic cohort I was providing care to was part of what many refer to as the Silent Generation. Born between 1925 and 1945, the Silent Generation are known for their "waste not, want not" mentality that many suggest they learned from living through the Great Depression. They are a population of fifty-five million in the US, and for the past twenty years had made up the majority of retirees.[4] They also gave birth to the Baby Boomers and, as they've gotten older, have been cared for by Boomers, who are an entirely different group of individuals.

The Baby Boomers were born between 1946 and 1964, and they are the largest generational cohort, making up 28 percent of the American population at seventy-six million people. Unlike their parents before them, the Boomers are known for their individualistic mindsets, are socially conscious, and make up the most substantial subset of the workforce. In 2011, the first wave of Boomers turned sixty-five, and it is projected that every day until 2030, ten thousand Baby Boomers will reach the age of retirement.[5] Over the fifteen years I've worked in senior

---

4   University of Missouri Extension, *Silent Generation / Traditionalists (born before 1946)*, n.d. http://extension.missouri.edu/extcouncil/documents/ecyl/meet-the-generations.pdf

5   University of Missouri Extension, *Baby Boomers (born 1946–1964)*, n.d. http://extension.missouri.edu/extcouncil/documents/ecyl/meet-the-generations.pdf

living, I've watched as the Boomers started to move into long-term care and witnessed the challenges the field has already begun to face as others attempt to care for such a large subset of the population.

For now, many Boomers still provide care to their parents of the Silent Generation, and they are doing so as they plan for their own future care needs. One of the biggest questions we ask in the field is, who will take care of the Boomers when they need it? So far, many in this demographic have been vocal about not wanting the same kinds of care their parents had, and they are working to change the "face" of old age by challenging stereotypes. But, as a whole, this group is still not planning for their long-term care needs, and, if we as a society are to provide care to such a large group of people effectively, it is important that this generation join the conversation and take responsibility for making a plan for their future care needs.

As the number of people in need of care grows, there is a significant decline in available caregivers, and reports of nursing homes being short-staffed continue to increase. Simultaneously, the number of family caregivers has increased, and the National Alliance on Caregiving and AARP report that there are 43.5 million unpaid caregivers in the US and that this number will continue to rise.[6] At such high numbers, family caregivers, particularly those of the Baby Boomer generation, will be the most affected by the burden of care. To become involved as someone's caregiver is a significant undertaking that involves a variety of factors, including your financial capability. Caregiving for an older adult is not a straightforward process, and there will be times when you have to handle vital decisions for the

---

6 National Alliance for Caregiving and AARP Public Policy Institute, *Caregiver Profile: The Millennial Caregiver* (Washington, DC: National Alliance for Caregiving and AARP Public Policy Institute, 2015), 6.

person in your care. To be put in this position without prior knowledge or understanding of the complexities of care is unfair and does not prepare you for the situations you will likely face along the way.

In this chapter, we take a closer look at the diversity of roles and settings that caregivers find themselves in, to shine light on the fact that caregivers take on many different roles, and, no matter what situation you find yourself in, you are never really alone in your journey. To recognize that people across our society are caregivers brings much-needed awareness of the support and flexibility we should be providing this growing subset of our population. As you move through this book, consider what kinds of care you feel comfortable with and able to provide your loved one.

Caregivers in the Home

There are family members who are willing and able to take in their loved ones who are living with dementia or may no longer be able to live independently. The multigenerational home (grandparents, parents, and children living in the same household) is a growing trend in our society. Pew Research estimates that sixty-four million people live in multigenerational homes, and this number will continue to rise as children move back home after college to save money and older adults move in to save on expenses or seek care.[7]

---

7 D'vera Cohn and Jeffrey S. Passel, "A record 64 million Americans live in multigenerational households," Pew Research Center, April 5, 2018, accessed April 1, 2019, http://www.pewresearch.org/fact-tank/2018/04/05/a-record-64-million-americans-live-in-multigenerational-households/.

There are many benefits to living together and, while there are challenges, many such caregivers feel reassured that, if anything were to happen, they would be right there to help. There is more time to get to know and support your loved one during this new phase of their life. Coming together for mealtimes or spending quality time watching a movie or playing a game creates lasting memories you can look back on and cherish.

It is also easier to establish and maintain a caregiving routine when you live together. Particularly when you care for someone living with Alzheimer's disease or dementia, following a routine will aid in making each task a bit smoother. Living together can even help save the family money if your loved one is willing and able to contribute to the household. However, while it may sound economically savvy to invite your loved one to live with you, the decision shouldn't be made lightly.

The traditional single-family home was designed for the thirty-something family, which means it is ill-equipped to support the needs of an older adult. Smaller doorways, two-story homes, tubs, and even doorknobs can become obstacles for older adults who have mobility issues or arthritis. When a family caregiver invites a loved one to live with them, they will most likely need to consider renovations and home safety modifications throughout the home. For some, the financial undertaking to make these changes may not be an issue, and, in fact, these kinds of universal design features will allow the family to grow in the home, too. But the economics of it all should be considered, as these elements will cost money and raise the question of who will pay for them.

Caregivers in the home also have little to no separation from their caregiving duties. Because they are in such close proximity, they become the default person for almost every situation, which in theory makes sense. Many times, I've heard caregivers express that they would rather be right there if something should happen; however, caregiving involves more than just emergency situations. If your loved one wakes up twenty times throughout the night to go to the bathroom and gets lost on the way back to their bedroom and becomes anxious and fearful, you are the person that will be getting up with them to take them back to their room and soothe their anxiety every time. You also will have to get up the next day and be able to function properly and be productive at your day job as if you hadn't just spent the night tired and anxious yourself.

It is in these raw caregiving moments that light needs to be shined on the fact that caregiving in the home is a 24/7 job. It can be traumatizing to watch your parent or loved one forget where the bathroom is, struggle to remember who you are while they are living under your roof, or yell at you for not helping them when that is all you are trying to do. It becomes so difficult to separate the parent from the diagnosis, and it is an unfair situation for any family member to have to face.

Yes, cohabiting can be the ideal situation for some families and, after a thoughtful conversation on boundaries and expectations, it most certainly can be beneficial. However, the decision to have your loved one move in with you may not be the best one simply because it makes the most economic or logistical sense or because it is the "right" thing to do. I urge you to take time to consider your options and your ability to be a caregiver at all times, throughout the day and night. Take comfort in knowing it's okay to decide that co-living is not the best choice for you, your loved one, and your family.

Caregivers with a Loved One in a Nursing Home

Caregivers with a loved one living in a nursing home have a vital role in the care and well-being of their loved one. They may not realize it, but their presence ensures the safety of their loved one and ensures that the care that they are receiving is not the only thing they have to look forward to. They can count on you as a familiar face to remind them that they are more than their care needs—that they are still able to live a life beyond the assistance of daily living they receive from their caregivers. This break from the constant medical focus is a breath of fresh air for so many individuals who have no other choice than to move into a care home.

A person's ability to engage with their loved ones while in the care of professionals is essential to their quality of life and their well-being. Residents who do not have any visitors struggle to find companionship while living in a nursing home. Yes, there are people there every day to take care of them, but they are paid. While they are willing and may even create bonds with these individuals, they are there to fulfill their duties and, if they have to leave, will do so despite these bonds. Family members play a significant role in the safety and well-being of their loved ones living in a nursing home; they are still needed and are still caregivers, even if the care recipient is living in a nursing home. Too many family members entrust companionship to the caregivers they or their loved ones are paying to take care of them. It is possible that the sight of their loved one in need of such skilled care is just too much to handle for some, and they may stop coming altogether. But they need you now more than ever.

Transitioning into a care home is a new chapter in someone's life, but that does not have to mean it is the last. A lot of learning happens in these settings. People learn how they handle giving up control of many of their normal functions, and they entrust those around them to provide for them in a way that they have spent most of their life doing on their own. For family members, it is hard to see this, to look past the glaring realities of your loved one's health or even cognitive decline. They will change reasonably quickly while they are here, but that doesn't mean you shouldn't be able to try to get to know them as they maneuver through this process. You are and always will be an important part of their lives, and to not be there during this frightening period can cause profound regret as the loved one passes away. You are their family first, and you deserve the chance to embrace this role and to help guide them through this new phase.

The Long-Distance Caregiver

A long-distance caregiver is someone who lives at least an hour away from the person in need of care—someone who is not able to pop over at a moment's notice and often needs coordination to make a trip over to the individual's home. Generally, long-distance caregivers are not the primary caregiver, and will often act as the support to the family member living closer to the care recipient. It is challenging for someone who lives far away to know how they can meaningfully engage in their loved one's care, but there are ways to play a significant role even if it means that you are a just a little bit more hands-off in your approach.

If you are a long-distance caregiver, knowing how you can help and where you should start in the caregiving process can be difficult. Start by having a conversation with your loved one and their primary caregiver (if this is someone other than you). They will both have a better sense of how you can be most helpful and this will prevent you jumping into, and perhaps disrupting, an already well-established process.

A long-distance caregiver has an excellent opportunity to be much-needed support for the primary caregiver in their loved one's life. The daily tasks of caregiving are draining, so taking the administrative to-dos from their list can sometimes save them both time and energy that they can refocus on themselves or the care recipient. The times when you do come into town can provide respite breaks for the primary caregiver, and you should include them in your plans for your trip home so they can schedule their time accordingly.

Researching and knowing the resources in your loved one's community is another great way to support them from afar. You may not be able to ensure they are exercising daily, but you can work to coordinate their attendance at their local senior center in hopes they exercise there! Checking out their local Area Agency on Aging is a great place to start in your community resource search—the AoA no doubt has already done most of the research and can point you in the right direction if you are looking for something specific for your loved one.

There is a lot of support and help that a long-distance caregiver can provide without physically being with their loved one. Technology has done a great deal to expand the role of the long-distance caregiver, too. For example, my next-door neighbor grocery-shops for her mom who lives out West and has the groceries delivered to her front door, so her mom doesn't have to worry about going on her own. Online bill pay is another way long-distance caregivers can use technology to support their loved one.

In addition to the practical support that technology can help you provide, opportunities for emotional connection and relationship-building have increased as well. For instance, platforms like Skype or Facetime are fun ways to connect and interact with them that allow them to see you as you talk. You can also send home movies of yourself and your family that will help keep them engaged and present in your life with them. If your loved one has Alzheimer's disease or other forms of dementia, you can create videos or a playlist of their favorite sing-along songs. Finding ways to engage with them through technology is a close alternative to being there in person when you live too far away to visit.

Caregivers in the Workplace

I have worked in a variety of settings, but I always seem to encounter a coworker who is also a family caregiver. When I tell them my focus in the aging field, our conversations can quickly become personal. These deeply personal stories of caregiving are becoming more frequent in the workplace. And for these workers, strain from outside stressors undoubtedly has an impact on their productivity and performance. AARP reports that 61 percent of family caregivers are currently employed either full-time or part-time.[8] Since this number will only increase in the coming years, this issue demands attention.

---

8   Lynn Feinberg and Rita Choula, "Understanding the Impact of Family Caregiving on Work," Fact Sheet 271, AARP Public Policy Institute, October 2012, accessed April 1, 2019, http://www.aarp.org/content/dam/aarp/research/public_policy_institute/ltc/2012/understanding-impact-family-caregiving-work-AARP-ppi-ltc.pdf.

For instance, one past coworker, although she made a decent living wage, was concerned that her parents, who never saved for retirement, would be retiring just as her second daughter started college. Since she was responsible for paying for both, she half-humorously joked that she had come to realize she will never be able to afford to retire. Another example happened on the way to lunch the other day. I walked by a woman noticeably upset at the sudden aphasia (a language disorder that affects a person's speech) her father was experiencing after a recent stroke. She expressed frustration at her inability to understand him, sadness that her father was ill, and exhaustion that now, on top of preparing her kids for a new school year, she would be spending the next few months searching for care facilities. In both cases, and the countless others I have encountered, there is a noticeable trend. As they are speaking, a look of disbelief is in their eyes, a shocked tone is in their voice, and a declarative "I don't know how I'm going to do it" is said at the end of each story.

Advocates for caregivers push companies to realize the importance of understanding and planning for a workforce made up of family caregivers. And for a good reason: without flexibility and understanding from businesses, caregivers are faced with having to leave the workforce altogether to support the needs of the older adult in their life. Early retirement then puts a strain on their ability to afford their own future care needs.

What Can Employers Do?

First, companies need to accept that this is a workplace issue. They will find that there is a range of policies and programs they can adopt to better support their workforce.

Hold a meeting. You may already have a weekly meeting on the calendar. Take five minutes to announce interest in this initiative, and possibly even to survey how many of the employees are in fact caregivers.

Collect and distribute caregiving resources. AARP is a national leader in advocating for caregivers. Their program ReACT is an online resource designed for the workplace which acquaints employers with best practices to support their workforce and maintain productivity.[9]

Start a workgroup. Opportunities for employees to meet and discuss shared experiences can do wonders for their mental health. Although this meeting could be held before or after business hours, holding it during office hours ensures that all employees can attend if they want to.

Consider telework and compensatory time. The typical nine-to-five workday is confining and offers little opportunity to schedule medical appointments for our loved ones without having to take time off work. Teleworking and comp time provide flexibility and allow employees to attend appointments while maintaining productivity.

Investing in staff creates a friendlier and more productive workforce. There are a staggering number of caregivers with full-time and part-time jobs, and the number will only increase over the next few years. Employers have an opportunity to not only foster a healthy work environment within their company, but also provide a better quality of life for their employees and, in turn, the older adults who depend on them every day.

---

9 Respect a Caregiver's Time Coalition (ReACT) and AARP, *Supporting Working Caregivers: Case Studies of Promising Practices,* Respect a Caregiver's Time Coalition (ReACT) and AARP, June 2017, accessed April 1, 2019, http://respectcaregivers.org/wp-content/uploads/2017/05/AARP-ReAct-MASTER-web.pdf.

The Sandwich Generation

An individual considered part of the Sandwich Generation has a parent over sixty-five and a child under eighteen or a grown child still in need of parental support. Pew Research found that 71 percent are aged forty to fifty-nine and are providing care at both ends of the spectrum at the same time. For many years, Baby Boomers made up the bulk of the Sandwich Generation; however, as Baby Boomers continue to age, they are now being cared for by the next generation of the Sandwiched—Gen X who were born between 1965 and 1979 and are currently between thirty-nine and fifty-three years old.[10]

The Sandwich Generation makes up the bulk of our workforce, and, while more affluent households ($100,000 a year or more) are more likely to provide this type of care, the Sandwich phenomenon does not discriminate. This generation reports providing care, financial support, and emotional support to both their children and their parents simultaneously. A majority also feel just as obligated to provide for their aging parents during this phase of their life as they do to provide for their children.[11]

Becoming a caregiver to both parents and children in midlife offers a unique perspective on the spectrum of life. Some caregivers find it humbling and a great honor to be able to provide this kind of love and support to their family. This is a beautiful sentiment that is unique in the caregiving experience, as many of these individuals will learn how to provide care on a variety of levels. However, the financial burden of

---

10 Kim Parker and Eileen Patten, *The Sandwich Generation Rising Financial Burdens for Middle-Aged Americans* (Washington, DC: Pew Research Center Social and Demographic Trends, 2013).

11 Ibid.

providing for both children and parents is great, especially as caregivers try to save for retirement. On average, the Sandwich Generation will spend seven thousand dollars in out-of-pocket caregiving costs.[12]

The Millennial Caregiver

I am a Millennial. I am right on the cusp of the generational shift, and, over the past couple of years, I've noticed a distinct change in the conversations I have with others in my cohort. While we discuss near-future decisions like careers, homes, and starting a family, the question of how close to home we should stay becomes a critical factor in the decision-making process. Why wouldn't it? The comforts of home are attractive to many of us, especially as we get a bit older and feel more inclined to carry on family traditions. Being closer to home also helps if and when close family members start to need additional care or support.

The National Alliance for Caregiving and AARP Public Policy Institute's report on the Millennial Caregivers says the average age of this cohort's caregiver is twenty-seven. They are working full-time, half of them live with a spouse or partner, and on average they have graduated high school and taken some college courses. All live with or live close to the care recipient.[13]

---

12   Jody Gasfriend, "Survival for the Sandwich Generation: Navigating the Hidden Costs for Working Caregivers," *Salon*, May 21, 2018, accessed April 1, 2019, https://www.salon.com/2018/05/20/surviving-the-sandwich-generation-navigating-hidden-costs-for-the-working-caregiver/.

13   National Alliance for Caregiving and AARP Public Policy Institute, "Caregiving in the U.S. 2015," June 2015, accessed April 1, 2019, https://www.caregiving.org/wp-content/uploads/2015/05/2015_CaregivingintheUS_Final-Report-June-4_WEB.pdf.

For those who aren't yet caregivers, the chances of becoming one are incredibly high due to the number of older adults who will be in need of care over the next twenty years. An increased generational focus on higher education and career means that many in the Millennial cohort will start a family and buy a home much later than their parents did. A later start means they will be in full-blown parenting and career mode when their parents begin to need additional care. Many of them are already privy to the realities of the family caregiver role. Their parents are Baby Boomers who have had the wild experience of raising a new generation while caring for the one that came before them. They are now left with the question, "Who's going to take care of me?"

The Caregiver for the Caregiver

Many caregivers are so busy taking care of their parent or loved one that they have either forgotten to or chosen not to take care of themselves, leaving their spouses, children, other family members, and even friends to step up and help take care of the caregiver's needs.

While this attention may not be as physically demanding as what the caregiver is providing for the older adult, these assistants to the caregiver work in several other ways. They provide emotional support and will spend most of their time listening and allowing the caregiver a safe space to vent. They assist in researching resources and support networks in the community. They understand their time with the person will change due to the scheduling constraints that accompany caregiving demands.

The assistant to the caregiver will most likely see it all and provide the bulk of the emotional support without receiving much reciprocation. Caregivers will spend all their time and energy on their loved one's care so that, too often, they have little left to give to other loved ones in their lives. It can be challenging to strike a balance when in the throes of caregiving, but the support you are providing them does not go unnoticed.

It Takes a Village

Caregivers are our neighbors, our coworkers, our friends, and our families. They carry on each day with the needs of their families and their loved ones on their minds. Caregivers are a part of the fabric of our society, which is essential to acknowledge for two reasons: 1) You, the caregiver, have representation and validation that you are not alone in this journey, and 2) our society sees the needs of our caregivers and can provide them with structural support. Caregiving needs are wide-ranging and rapidly changing today, and government agencies, businesses, non-profit organizations, and community members not only recognize these needs and changes but also are in the process of changing the way they do business and offering a host of resources and services for our care recipients.

I heard a recent news story about a small-town family whose son uses a wheelchair. Their community park installed a wheelchair-accessible swing, and the mom made a comment that resonated. She said it had been mainly up to the family to make the world available for her son, which meant everything from walking/ wheeling down the street to recreational pursuits so her son could have a fun childhood. An image of her son and the rest of the family laughing and smiling around the swing set spoke strongly of the joy that this intervention had brought to this family. Because this community chose to install an accessible swing, this mother didn't have to explain to her son why he couldn't play in the park like all the other kids. She didn't have to figure out another way to have fun outdoors with her family. Because the town took the initiative to provide the structural support, she didn't have to adapt and could enjoy a playful moment with her son.

While this example speaks to the needs of a younger generation, I believe the situation is the same for older adults as well. Our communities and businesses have an excellent opportunity to design for the needs of older adults because, when you plan for them, you benefit everyone in the community. Efficiently designing for older adults requires design thinking because it is crucial that thought, empathy, and emotion are incorporated into the design. An efficient design will allow an older adult to continue to age independently and help them feel safe and secure in their surroundings.

Making the transition to an age-friendly community can be a process. However, there are relatively small-scale design features a city can implement to get the innovation process started. Like the accessible wheelchair swing, brightly painted crosswalks, wheelchair access on every street corner, and handrails along walkways are just minor changes communities can make to keep older adults and their caregivers active in their community. Caregivers, too, can play an active role in the shift in design for our communities. If your loved one needs a wheelchair ramp on their street corner, then consider calling your neighborhood associations or advocating on their behalf at your local town hall meetings. Notifying community organizations, businesses, government, etc. of the specific needs is the fastest way to see changes.

Over the past fifteen years I've witnessed a shift in this direction—a shift that recognizes the needs of caregivers and offers support to help you provide the best care to older adults. There are resources and people out there advocating on your behalf and I am encouraged by the progress, but we aren't all the way there yet. Not all communities offer fair pricing for adult day services or respite care, and we haven't really talked about caregiving on a personal one-on-one level. There are ways to maintain other relationships while caregiving, and it is okay to say you can't provide care today.

As an activities professional, I worked with individuals living with Alzheimer's disease or other forms of dementia on a daily basis. I had to learn non-medical ways to intervene for each when they started to become upset or anxious. Designing a caregiving plan that would benefit the individual while reducing my stress and worry about them was essential to my ability to provide a good quality of care and a good quality of life to each resident. Over time, I learned what worked and what didn't work, and I soon had many tools in my "arsenal" for each resident I worked with. These tools are what you, the family caregiver, are left to figure out on your own; as you play many different roles, like nurse, aide, dietitian, and transportation and recreation provider, it is nearly impossible to create a cohesive caregiving plan.

You are caring for someone you've known for some time; they know you and trust you. You have memories with them that have created a foundation for the caregiving process. But your relationship with them shouldn't have to take the back seat. Activities provide a fantastic opportunity to refocus your attention on the relationship with your loved one, and thus make the caregiving experience more manageable and less stressful.

As you continue on your caregiving journey, it is important to recognize that you are not alone, and that there are resources and connections available to ensure that you are able to provide the best quality of care to your loved one. Don't be afraid to explore your boundaries and decide for yourself what type of care you can provide on your own, and where you may need additional support.

Chapter Two

Three Ways to Avoid Caregiver Burnout

No matter how you became a caregiver, the job has specific characteristics. It will require your full attention. It will take all of your emotional capacity. You will have to watch as your loved one declines in health and capability, but you will also be witness to a beautiful transition in the human life cycle. I've often equated the aging process to that of a butterfly. We traditionally view old age as a deterioration of life, but, honestly, it is not—the amount of love and laughter that older adults have still brings me a smile when I'm feeling down. Or worrying about my age. Despite being told that our later years are filled with decline and loss of independence, these individuals find a way to live life to the fullest and to find humor in even the darkest of times.

How does this help a caregiver? The general fear that our elders are actively transitioning from this life is a constant in the mind of a caregiver. This future mindset rips away opportunities to be in the moment with yourself and to grapple with the emotions you are experiencing. You are left to move through the motions without ever truly being given the chance to express how the caregiving is making you feel. Providing care to another person is a sacrifice, and it takes time to process everything you are witnessing, feeling, and doing. These are your loved ones. These are people you have spent time with, have built memories with, and who have no doubt taught you many of the things you know today.

Such an intense experience as a caregiver can wear on your emotions and even on your ability to provide quality care for the duration of the recipient's life. You need to take breaks from caregiving periodically, or you will get burned out. Many caregivers interpret the general stress and tiredness they feel as just another symptom of a hectic, day-to-day life. We are used to working long hours and making up for that time with a two-week vacation each year. While a holiday helps, two weeks away won't be enough to prevent caregiver burnout. Identifying symptoms of exhaustion and incorporating a self-care routine are essential skills caregivers should develop, especially if they are expected to provide high levels of care over a long period of time.

What Is Caregiver Burnout?

Caregiving doesn't have normal business hours, has no concept of vacation days, sick days, or personal days, and occurs 24/7, whether you are asleep or awake. To raise a family, go to work, and manage finances, all while providing care to a loved one, leaves you with little time to spend on yourself. But to purposefully take time to slow down is exactly what you need to be able to handle all the responsibilities in your life. To expend all your energy without recharging will cause emotional, mental, and physical exhaustion. When prolonged, this exhaustion can lead to resentment or anger, poor self-care and caregiving, depression, stress, and anxiety, all of which will inhibit your ability to manage all your responsibilities.

The Alzheimer's Association identifies ten symptoms of caregiver stress[14]:

1. Denial about the disease and its effect on the person who has been diagnosed.

2. Anger at the person with Alzheimer's or frustration that they can't do the things they used to be able to do.

3. Withdrawal from friends and activities that used to make you feel good.

4. Anxiety about the future and facing another day.

5. Depression that breaks your spirit and affects your ability to cope.

6. Exhaustion that makes it nearly impossible to complete necessary daily tasks.

7. Sleeplessness caused by a never-ending list of concerns.

8. Irritability that leads to moodiness and triggers negative responses and actions.

9. Lack of concentration that makes it difficult to perform familiar tasks.

10. Health problems that begin to take a mental and physical toll.

It is hard to distinguish between yourself and your role as a caregiver because providing care to another person who needs you in such an intimate way forms a strong connection between the two of you. To step away from that role to take care of yourself can cause feelings of guilt, so many choose not

---

14 Alzheimer's Association, "Caregiver Stress," Alzheimer's Association, n.d., accessed April 1, 2019, https://www.alz.org/help-support/caregiving/caregiver-health/caregiver-stress

to, and continue to provide care even though they are too tired or stressed to do so correctly. This chapter will go over three main ways you can avoid caregiver burnout: 1) self-care, 2) find a support network, and 3) don't just focus on your loved one's physical well-being. Incorporating these ideas into your daily routine should make the experience less stressful on you, and even offers time within the regular hectic schedule to have some fun together!

Focus on Self-Care

In the midst of caregiving, it is understandably difficult to find a personal moment to spare for yourself. To do this may even require a drastic shift in your daily routine—a routine that, while hectic, provides the predictability and repetition needed to accomplish all the necessary daily tasks. The role of caregiver will require your full attention. Between activities of daily living, medication management, doctor's appointments, and mealtimes, there isn't time left to do much of anything else. Whether a family member or not, providing this type of care will leave a person quickly feeling burned out.

And yes, "take care of yourself" is an all-too-common piece of advice which I am sure you have heard before. What I mean is that taking care of the self goes beyond occasionally treating yourself to a spa day. You deserve credit and validation that what you are doing is hard work. That providing care is sometimes a thankless job, and the care decisions you make for another person are difficult. As humans, we deserve to spend time on ourselves—time to reflect on the progress we have made in our lives, the experiences we have endured, and the relationships we have cultivated along the way.

Validation of the hard work you are putting into the care of your loved one may not always come from those around you. It is difficult for those on the outside to ever truly understand what you are going through. Giving yourself gentle reminders throughout the day can offer self-assurance that you are doing the best you can to provide the best quality of life for your loved one.

Repeat these affirmations daily:

"I am a good person."

"I am lightening my load."

"I take care of the world when I take care of myself."

"I am worth taking time for."

"I have the right to my own time beyond taking care of others."

Only you have control of where your energy is spent, and while, yes, situations often feel outside of our control, the time and effort you spend thinking positively or negatively about any one circumstance is entirely your own. Becoming mindful of how you spend your time is extremely important. Our societal values about hard work often leave little time for much else. Take back control of your own time and invest your energy in things that will make you feel good. You are allowed to be happy, and you are allowed to take care of yourself.

You may not even know how or where to begin with the self-care process. I've talked with many caregivers who until then had never thought twice about how they spent their time because simple things, like watching a favorite TV show or a night out with girlfriends, were all they needed to de-stress from their workday. Health experts will report to us the things we should do for self-care, like eat healthily or exercise daily, but if you are being told you have to do these things, it seems more like an obligation than an investment in personal well-being.

Identify Your Values

Recently I was struggling with my career choices. I hated the idea of working in an environment that saw me as just another cog in the wheel. I didn't want to have an anxiety attack every time I had to miss a day of work for a routine doctor's appointment, or come home each day exhausted from the demands of the job. I was too early in my career to have to spend the next thirty years or so unhappy.

In a bit of half-hearted research, I came across a YouTube video on creating a "Values List." I thought it was an interesting idea, and six months later I finally got around to building my list. I focused on the fundamental things I wanted in a prospective employer and my potential role in that job.

Relaxed, autonomous, community-focused, kind, and respectful were all words I put down on my page. I wrote out twenty more words or so, and then honed in on the eight that I felt represented my values the most. At the end of the exercise, I felt validated and empowered to continue my job search with these values in mind. I was amazed that, within a month of writing out this list, I landed my dream job, working in the community with a group of kind and respectful colleagues who have welcomed me and shown me there is a way to work in my field of choice without feeling burned out at the end of each day.

Writing a values list can sound more like a time-waster than a time-saver. I say this because that is exactly how I perceived the exercise, too. I write from my own example because, during this time of my life, it seemed like I had no control over my career circumstances. Because I needed to pay my bills and put food on the table, I felt forced to take the first job that came down the pike. Understanding my values changed this.

As a family caregiver, you may find yourself in an impossible situation, because your loved one needs you (like, really needs you) and you have a lifestyle that you need to sustain. You may believe the only option is to maintain the hectic day-to-day pattern you have found yourself in. To understand how you want to spend your time and what you want to prioritize is hugely empowering and allows you to make decisions that seek to benefit you and not just the meet the circumstances in which you find yourself. Granted, you may find you need to make compromises; mine was a lower salary and an entry-level position, but the time and peace of mind is well worth it!

Values List

Directions: Grab a pencil or pen, set a timer for twenty minutes, find a quiet and comfortable seat, and then spend a few moments brainstorming. Write down twenty personal values you identify with most.

1. _____

2. _____

3. _____

4. _____

5. _____

6. _____

7. _____

8. _____

9. _____

10. _____

11. _____

12. _____

13. _____

14. _____

15. _____

16. _____

17. _____

18. _____

19. _____

20. _____

Values List

Directions: Out of the 20 you wrote down re-write the 8 that you want to reflect on in your everyday.

1. _____

2. _____

3. _____

4. _____

5. _____

6. _____

7. _____

8. _____

Values Word List

The list below is just to get you started you can put down any word that means something to you.

Achievement	Serenity	Certainty	Affection	Giving	Fitness	Respect
Freedom	Enjoyment	Wealth	Kindness	Simplicity	Charm	Sensitivity
Dependability	Guidance	Diversity	Faith	Balance	Enthusiasm	Tradition
Health	Cheerfulness	Joy	Originality	Passion	Gratefulness	Vitality
Integrity	Friendliness	Humor	Boldness	Fairness	Adaptability	Independence
Belongingness	Harmony	Adventure	Wisdom	Leadership	Happiness	Warmth
Inspiration	Determination	Growth	Honesty	Peacefulness	Delight	Love
Calmness	Imagination	Efficiency	Motivation	Ambition	Fun	Zest

Find a Support Network

Providing care for a family member can feel overwhelming, and even lonely at times. It's not like you had ample amounts of free time before assuming this role. A work/life balance is an eternal human debate, and we have all felt the pressure at some point to gracefully manage the responsibilities of both.

For family caregivers, the luxury of grace is often too far from reality to even daydream about. The average family caregiver of an older adult in America is a forty-nine-year-old female.[15] Too young to retire and still raising a family, these individuals/ parents/workers/caregivers are left to "figure it out" when it comes to balancing all their responsibilities.

The stresses that come with caregiving are unique and can cause a range of thoughts and feelings that you can't believe you are actually having. Joining a group or network of people that are caregiving for a loved one will validate your experience and help with any negative thoughts you may be having as a result. Fortunately, the progress of technology has made finding resources and support networks easier. There are plenty of written materials about caring for older adults, but a growing trend is the number of support groups and caregiving communities popping up all over the web. These platforms allow you to easily join and chat with hundreds of people who are experiencing the same frustrations, and even have the same questions, as you.

Caregiving topics are wide-ranging, and it is easy to get lost and even confused by the sheer amount of information out there on the internet. To start your search, be sure to hone in on key words or topics you are seeking advice about; for example, a simple search on "dementia" resulted in ninety-two million results on Google. Instead, use key phrases such as "coping with dementia" or "online caregiver support groups" that will yield results on specific articles or websites that offer this type of targeted information.

Reliable sources will have their logo and name clearly displayed on their page, and the About page will explain the mission or

---

15 Feinberg and Choula, "Understanding the Impact of Family Caregiving on Work." https:// www.aarp.org/content/dam/aarp/research/public_policy_institute/ltc/2012/understanding-impact-family-caregiving-work-AARP-ppi-ltc.pdf.

purpose for providing information. Also, be sure to check the dates on the articles posted. If a page is active, the information is more likely to be current. Avoid websites with a ton of advertisements, even if the content is good; they are more likely trying to sell you a product than to offer you sage advice. If you still aren't sure, check to see if they have a social media following on Facebook, Twitter, or Instagram and read the comments from other subscribers to see how helpful they are to others.

The next section offers a targeted group of resources I either have worked with personally or have found to be the most helpful over the years.

Books and Blogs

The AlzAuthors

The AlzAuthors was created and is now run by five incredible women: Ann Campanella, Vicki Tapia, Jean Lee, Kathryn Harrison, and Marianne Sciucco.

Their mission is to share both their own and others' experiences to bring knowledge, comfort, and understanding to others on this caregiving journey. Their books were written with a common goal: To make a difference![16]

They have gathered and shared over a hundred book authors and blog writers on their website, www.alzauthors.com, who share their personal experiences with Alzheimer's to ease the path for others.

---

16   AlzAuthors, last modified 2019. https://www.alzauthors.com.

Carol Bradley Bursack, *Minding Our Elders*

I was thrilled when Carol agreed to write the foreword to this book. Her experience in providing care to seven people is unparalleled by any caregiving story I've ever heard. Her book, *Minding Our Elders*, shares personal stories from various backgrounds, and serves as a portable support group for caregivers in many situations.[17]

National and International Organizations

The Family Caregiver Alliance, National Center on Aging

The FCA is a non-profit whose mission is to improve the quality of life for caregivers and those they care for through information, services, and advocacy. They have gathered a series of articles and programs designed to help the family caregiver on their website, www.caregiver.org.

The National Center on Aging has developed profiles for all fifty states and stays current on policy and legislation that affects caregivers and their loved ones. Their Caregiver Connect program offers an unmoderated online support group for families, partners, and other caregivers of adults with disorders such as Alzheimer's, stroke, brain injury, and other chronic debilitating health conditions. The group offers a safe place to discuss the stresses, challenges, and rewards of providing care for a loved one.[18]

---

17 Carol Bradley Bursack, *Minding our Elders*, last modified 2019. https://mindingourelders.com.

18 Family Caregiver Alliance, last modified 2019, https://www.caregiver.org.

The National Consumer Voice

The National Consumer Voice is the leading national voice representing consumers in issues related to long-term care, helping ensure that consumers are empowered to advocate for themselves. They are a primary source of information and tools for consumers, families, caregivers, advocates, and ombudsmen to help ensure quality care for the individual.

Their website is easy to navigate and aims to help educate and support families with loved ones living in long-term care settings. Their work seeks to empower both individuals residing in care homes and their loved ones to stay safe and protected in the long-term care setting of their choice.[19]

The International Alliance of Carer Organizations

The IACO is an offshoot of the National Alliance of Caregiving Organizations, and its mission is to build a strong international network of carer organizations to share ideas, programs, and research that can bring visibility and support to family caregivers around the globe.[20]

Informal Support Groups

Facebook

Facebook has a number of support groups that were started by caregivers. These groups range in focus from caregivers providing dementia care to caregivers who are still raising

---

19 The National Consumer Voice, last modified 2019. https://theconsumervoice.org.

20 International Alliance of Carer Organizations (IACO), last modified 2019. https:// internationalcarers.org/.

children. Searching for caregiver support groups will yield a variety of options for you to peruse and join at your leisure.

Local Meet-Ups

Local meet-up groups are popping up all over the country. Search for local meet-up groups or for a local Facebook group if meeting in person is preferred.

Dementia Mentors

Dementia Mentors offers support to individuals after a diagnosis of dementia and is a great resource to provide your loved one if they have been diagnosed with a form of dementia. The group meets online in its Virtual Memory Cafes, and support comes from others who have been diagnosed.[21] Their website is easy to navigate, and if you contact them and let them know what type of dementia you or your loved one has, they will match you with a mentor who has the same diagnosis. To learn more, check out their website, www.dementiamentors.org.

Finding the right support system for you and your situation is essential; the caregiver resources and groups listed here are a starting point. Take time to research caregivers who are already out there and eager to help point you in the right direction.

Exercise: Take twenty minutes to search online for caregiving support forums/blogs/books. Add the top five results of your search to your favorites so you can access them any time.

---

21 Dementia Mentors, last modified 2019. https://www.dementiamentors.org/.

Schedule Quality Time

Quality time is extremely important, both for you as the caregiver and for the person you are caring for. You should be spending quality time together and quality time apart. While the role of caregiver adds several extra tasks onto an already full to-do list, there are a few ways to make doing these things more meaningful.

Taking a break from caregiving duties is hard because caregiving is an identity and a role that you are always playing, even after your loved one passes away. Stepping back from your role may not be easy, but the time you spend not directly providing care can be. All you need to do is schedule this time and do meaningful activities within it. To be conscious of how you spend your time brings with it an enlightening experience that would otherwise be missed. Yes, time relaxing with a favorite TV show is nice, but the real value comes from moments of time that you've designed for yourself. The moments spent with or away from your loved one will be the times you remember the most when they have moved on, and it is then that you will want these moments back the most.

Spending Quality Time Together

Living in the moment is a common piece of advice. Working with individuals with dementia taught me this concept at a very young age. A moment of anger or frustration doesn't have to stay with you throughout your day and can be quickly turned around with a bit of friendly company. It was in these moments that I realized that those living with dementia are not gone. They are incredibly present. We just have to make the conscious effort to join them where they are.

As their caregiver, you will spend so much time thinking about their physical and medical well-being. A constant focus on this one aspect of your loved one's life makes it difficult to see them as anything more than a patient or an obligation. You know them beyond this role, and to engage with them in ways that are familiar and fun is the easiest way to enjoy your time together and refocus on why you are caregiving for them in the first place.

Activity pursuits are about more than just keeping someone entertained. The moments spent together, doing something you and your family member love to do, are the moments when you "find" them again. These moments are precious, and, for someone living with Alzheimer's disease or other forms of dementia, it is these times that matter the most.

There are five categories of engagement pursuits that are important to engage your loved one with, and they are:

1. Mental (trivia, reading)

2. Emotional (reminiscing, music)

3. Physical (exercise)

4. Spiritual (church, religious pursuits)

5. Social (spending time with others their age, friends, and family members)

Activities don't even have to be a big to-do. In fact, I often discourage elaborate activities because they will be too tiring and overstimulating for your loved one. Rather than elaborate activities, quiet, one-on-one activities like singing along to their favorite songs or having fun with trivia are a great way to stimulate their minds while having fun.

In the nursing home, we are equipped with an activities calendar, which acts as a guide for us to stay organized and offers these types of social pursuits in a way that is easy and manageable for residents and staff. As a family caregiver, taking time to create an activities calendar won't always be possible; however, if you keep in mind the five engagement pursuits and find ways to incorporate them, you'll see your loved one is more at ease and more engaged, which allows you the opportunity to spend quality time together.

Activities offer both you and your loved one a chance to slow down and spend time together in a meaningful way. Taking activity breaks throughout the day also gives you an opportunity to step away from being the caregiver and refocus on being the daughter, the son, the friend you've always been. These moments enhance the caregiving experience and help to release stress or anxiety that could otherwise lead to burnout.

A great activity idea that could help is a memory board, which captures a special moment or time period in someone's life by displaying pictures and mementos from that time and a brief description of each memory. Creating a memory board is a fun and meaningful activity that can be worked on whenever you have a spare moment to spend. A memory board allows you and your loved one to reminisce together, and, when complete, it offers a wonderful conversation piece for when friends and family members come over.

Memory Board Activity

To start this project, talk with your loved one about a possible theme. When I did this activity with the residents at one nursing home, a resident created a board for a childhood game she used to play with her sister, "Callsies." Her board had a drawing of two phones at the top, a picture of her and her sister, and directions on how they would play this make-believe game.

For example, if your loved one talks about their childhood home a lot, this activity will allow them to reminisce in a positive way.

Topic conversation starters:

- Where did you grow up?

- What was your favorite game as a kid?

- What was your favorite family vacation?

- What is your favorite family recipe?

Items you will need:

- One large poster board

- Scissors

- Glue

- Scrapbooking materials

- Family photos (that you don't mind cutting up and pasting)

- Mementos (concert tickets, hand-written family recipes)

- Magazines

- Markers or Sharpies

Directions:

- Choose a theme

- Sort through family photos and mementos together and choose the ones you want to use

- Gather materials and lay them out on the dining room table

- Start decorating the board together

- Write up a fun description of what the board represents and tape it to either the front or the back of the board so others can read it

- Once you are satisfied with the design, find a place to put it on display

A memory board activity satisfies the mental, social, and emotional engagement pursuit needs, but, more importantly, it carves out meaningful time to spend together, all while providing care.

Spending Quality Time Apart

Spending quality time apart is just as important as spending time together. This goes particularly for caregivers who live with or near the person they are taking care of. The primary family caregiver will spend more time with their loved one doing caregiving-related activities than they will doing fun engagement activities. Stepping away from your caregiving duties is not a bad thing. It is the healthiest thing for you to do as a caregiver, because providing intensive care without a break is the fastest way to burn yourself out. Both you and your loved one need a break from each other to maintain a healthy and prosperous care arrangement.

Your loved one may be entirely dependent on you for their care needs, but that doesn't necessarily mean they are happy with the idea of having to spend every free moment they have with you... and this goes for individuals living with dementia, too! Finding ways for your loved one to get out and socialize with people that aren't you will do wonders for the sanity of all involved!

The complexities of the caregiving process can easily cause socializing to sink to the bottom of your priorities list. But that doesn't mean your loved one should be stuck in their room watching TV. An often-overlooked benefit of moving into a long-term care option is the fact that residents in care homes have an abundance of social pursuits available to them throughout the day.

Understandably, it does take time to find ways for your loved one to socialize without you present. It's not like you can just drop them off at a restaurant and leave and, in many cases, it is for their safety and comfort that they have someone who can provide care for them nearby at all times.

Here are four ways to schedule time apart from your loved one:

1. Enlist the Help of Family and Friends

Don't be afraid to ask family and close friends for help. It may sound like an imposition, but it's often not. Family and friends are willing to help, but because caregiving is such a broad responsibility, it is hard for someone to know how to help. Do you need an hour to run to the grocery store? Invite a friend over to have coffee with your mom. It's just as much of a break for you as it is for the person you are providing care to! Plus, being around new people stimulates the mind and offers social interaction that those living with dementia or Alzheimer's disease desperately need.

2. Check Out Local Meet-Up Groups

In this age of technology, there are so many ways to meet new people and to find groups and clubs with like-minded people. As a caregiver, a local meet-up for caregivers may be a great way to meet people who know firsthand what you are going through. That, in and of itself, can be enough to provide the validation and time away you need to keep going.

Or, do you have a hobby that has fallen by the wayside since you've started caregiving? Finding a local meet-up that supports this hobby offers a great excuse to break away and to do something you enjoy. While you may have the caregiver title, that doesn't mean you aren't still in there somewhere. Take this as an opportunity to be YOU!

3. Senior Center or Adult Day Centers

There is always something going on at a senior center and, while not all are equipped to handle skilled care needs, they can be an excellent option for activity ideas and community resources that you and your loved one can tap into. Even if it is just for a couple of hours, your loved one can spend time away from you with people their age.

Adult day centers/adult day care/adult services are equipped to handle many skilled care needs and, while services vary, they are generally designed to meet the needs of older adults during the day while allowing them to continue to live with their families or in the community.

4. Respite Care

Caregivers are sometimes reluctant to seek professional help when they need a break from their caregiving duties. Most likely, the whole reason you became a full-time caregiver in the first place was that you didn't want someone else taking care of your loved one, right? It is not sustainable; even professional caregivers get burned out, and they get breaks and don't have the additional burden of emotional ties to the individual.

A great way to get a well-deserved break from caregiving and have some much-needed time to yourself is to seek out respite care for your loved one. Respite care is short-term living care for seniors, typically in an assisted living or memory care unit. Rather than moving into a room, your loved one will rent an apartment for a few weeks, and the staff takes over your duties while you take some well-deserved rest.

This is also an excellent opportunity for your loved one to be around new people. I've heard concerns from family members that their loved one wouldn't do well with the change to their routine. Care homes are probably the most regimented places out there, and, while your loved one may spend some time adjusting, they will no doubt adapt to the regular daily routine of the care home.

Step Back and Breathe

When you are in the midst of caregiving, it is easy to get caught up in day-to-day tasks without much conscious awareness of how you are feeling and how you are spending your time. You are focused on someone you love, and the fact that they entrusted their care to you speaks volumes about the love and respect that they hold for you. To hear this is important. You are stepping into a sacred role that will change you in ways you probably never thought could happen.

Each caregiving experience will be unique to your individual story and path, but that doesn't mean you should get lost along the way. Caregiver burnout can have a significant impact on your emotions, and many people express feelings of apathy and even anger toward the care recipient. While these emotions are real, they stem from the constant focus on ensuring your loved one is well-cared for and safe. These emotions aren't permanent and can be resolved if you take the time you need to be the family member or friend you've always been. Instead, consider these moments you have together, and build on the foundation of love and trust that the two of you have developed over the years. Time may be passing, but the moments you grab along the way will be some of the best you'll have.

Chapter Three
Dementia Care

There are many different levels of responsibility when it comes to dementia care. As a progressive disease with varying stages, a diagnosis of dementia is unique in the caregiving journey. Many people believe that a diagnosis of dementia somehow suggests that the person will immediately lose their function and memory capacity. While this may occur, it often doesn't happen until the individual is much older, and they will have many high-functioning years after a diagnosis.

Quite understandably, upon diagnosis, there will be feelings of doubt and uncertainties about your ability to care for your loved one. Dementia has developed a reputation for being "unreasonable" or draining, due to the various forms that it can grow into. All dementia behaviors are unique to the person. Although some symptoms may seem not to follow a pattern, over time you will learn that something is provoking a symptom, and your loved one is trying to explain this to you in the only way they know how.

Having worked primarily with individuals living with dementia, I know how common it is for caregivers to disengage from a person living with dementia. Professionals do this by calling residents by their diagnosis or room number, rather than their names. Both family members and professionals do this by talking about the person or answering questions for them, even though they are in the room. A diagnosis of dementia means many things and will require the individual and the caregiver to work together to relearn how to communicate with one another. It does not suggest that the individuals have lost the capacity to express themselves, only that the communication is going to occur differently.

There are noticeable patterns in the behaviors that present with dementia. Individual personality and life experiences will influence the way someone communicates, but generally they will respond and react in similar ways. These patterns have allowed many professionals to learn to use techniques like validation therapy or reminiscing as tools to soothe and redirect individuals who may be feeling especially anxious or even angry. Over time, you too will learn how your loved one is communicating with you. This chapter will outline ways to identify patterns and how to use these techniques to provide the best quality of care to your loved one.

The Language of Dementia

Dementia is a general term that often refers to a decline in cognitive ability. Dementia is not a normal part of aging. Because of its prevalence in older adults and our society's stereotypes about memory loss in old age, many people think of dementia as a part of the aging process.

Many people consider dementia a disease, but it is a group of symptoms. There are a number of different forms of dementia, and each has a unique set of traits. The most common types of dementia are:

- Alzheimer's disease

- Vascular dementia

- Dementia with Lewy bodies (DLB)

- Mixed dementia

- Parkinson's disease

- Frontotemporal dementia

- Creutzfeldt-Jakob disease

- Normal pressure hydrocephalus

- Huntington's disease

- Wernicke-Korsakoff syndrome

Each of these diagnoses has its own distinct set of needs. Approaches to delivering care will require adjustment based on individual assessment. Commonly, dementia affects a person's ability to communicate, and I mean communication in a broad sense. For instance, a person may still be able to speak, but the words they use don't make any sense to us, or maybe they are no longer able to use words and their words simply become sounds. A generalized perception of dementia causes many people to disregard conversation attempts from that individual, and if what they are saying to us isn't immediately apparent it is brushed off as a symptom of the diagnosis. Stereotypes have caused many to believe that the individual loses the ability to comprehend and appropriately interact with their environment.

The most common language patterns I've learned to pay attention to over the years are the use of intonation and facial expressions. It is my firm belief that individuals living with dementia are deliberate in their communication. We may not understand what they are trying to tell us, but that does not mean what they are trying to say doesn't make sense. The breakdown in communication between caregiver and care recipient affects how the caregiver both perceives and interacts with the individual with dementia. Again, language development will be different for everyone, but the ways we learn to understand can generally be the same. Below are three examples of how dementia affected a person's ability to speak, and how through investigation I was able to understand what they were trying to tell me.

An analogy I like to use to describe the miscommunication that occurs with those living with dementia is from a trip to Copenhagen I took with my husband. I was out for a walk in the city when this little dog came running up to me; I looked around for the owner and saw this woman approaching quickly behind the dog. I was hesitant to pet him because I was not able to communicate with his owner and didn't want to offend, so I just said hello to the pup without petting him. The woman then came up to me and started talking to me in Danish. I had no idea what she was saying, but I nodded and responded to what her tone or intonation was telling me, which was, "Why didn't you pet my dog?" When I didn't respond appropriately, she looked at me as if I was a bit off my rocker and walked away. I think about this instance a lot because she gave me the same look that many individuals living with dementia had when they came up to me and tried to tell me something that I couldn't understand. In both cases, it wasn't because the person wasn't making any sense; it was because I didn't understand the language they were using.

An example of how I've learned to listen to the tone of someone's voice while they speak, instead of trying to understand the words they are saying, is through my interactions with a resident I'll call Ms. Jones. Ms. Jones is a resident I used to work with and is a good example of how someone with dementia would communicate through their tone of voice. Ms. Jones would often come up to express her amusement about whatever it was she just witnessed. I could always tell because her hands would float up in the air as if she was conducting a choir. Her tone was light, and she would laugh and look to me to join her in her amusement, as if she were telling a joke or a funny story. Ms. Jones was no longer able to convey meaning through speech, but she could still communicate. By watching and interacting with Ms. Jones on a daily basis, I found that communication became easier and more fluent as I got to know her.

I also worked with Mr. Smith, who was diagnosed with aphasia. While he could still communicate with words, the words were jumbled and rarely "made sense" in the context of language. In conversation, Mr. Smith would join seemingly random words together, such as "the apple fell and whoops!" I started to notice that "apple" was a word he used a lot. To break it down further, apple was used a lot during certain times of the day. Over a few weeks, I started to realize that, to Mr. Smith, "apple" no longer represented a fruit, but instead held a larger contextual meaning of food or hunger.

In each of these examples, the individual with dementia continued to communicate with me as if I should understand every word they were telling me; they always believed they were clear. Their frustration escalated if I didn't understand what they were saying to me; as I was learning their language, I would often misunderstand. I found it particularly difficult to understand someone when they were upset and needed me to intervene in some way. I had to guess a lot of the time, and each time I was wrong, they knew I was wrong and would get more and more upset. At no point did it seem as though they believed they were at fault for the miscommunication. If they believe that they are speaking to us clearly, then that suggests that dementia does not take away their ability to appropriately respond to their environment or express themselves. It just takes away their ability to do so in the way that we have learned to understand.

As in any conversation, effective communication goes both ways, and as you are providing care to your loved one, it is crucial for you to be conscious of your tone and body language. I have found individuals living with dementia are quick to pick up on subtle changes in emotion, and can become defensive or even combative if they think you are angry or upset with them. For instance, if you are running late for work but still need to shower your loved one, you may rush through the care tasks, and while this helps you get the job done quicker, your loved one is more likely to put up a fight until you slow down.

The next section will discuss how to identify dementia triggers and how the use of all five senses will help you bridge the communication gap between you and your loved one, particularly for individuals who have aphasia or have become non-verbal due to dementia. An understanding of potential triggers, and methods to address the behaviors that are caused by the triggers, will allow you to pick up on patterns in the way they perceive things and respond to what is happening in their environment.

Dementia Triggers

Responding to the environment is part of our human evolution. We all use our senses to gauge both our internal and external function and safety. When we are hungry, we know because we feel a grumble in our stomach. If music or the TV is on too loud, we know to turn it down to a more comfortable level. We do this almost as second nature; often, we don't even realize we are doing it, partly because we have the autonomy to fix our discomfort before it gets overwhelming.

But have you ever had to wait a little longer to eat when you were already starving? Did this make you feel irritable and maybe even angry? And when you finally took that bite of food, those feelings of anger seemed to just melt away, didn't they?

I don't think this is much different for your loved one living with dementia. The only difference is that they are looking to you to fix the problem. They may not be able to tell you directly what is making them uneasy, and, more often than not, you will be faced with the triggered irritability rather than a direct statement like "I'm hungry" or "I'm cold." When you begin to view their "behaviors" as indicators rather than acts of hostility toward you, you'll begin to understand what they are trying to tell you.

People living with dementia are still human. Although that sounds like common sense, many people forget that these individuals have a range of emotions and are still affected by the same things we all are. Too often, medication is used to subdue an individual living with dementia because it is thought that their behaviors are a symptom of the disease rather than a response to their environment.

Drugs aren't a cure-all in dementia, and, while medication adherence is important, there are holistic ways to ease anxiety and anger for your loved one living with dementia. Dementia symptoms can be aggravated easily and will often make the individual highly sensitive to what is happening around them. The next section will focus on how you can pay close attention to certain sounds, smells, or sights within the room to help you home in on possible causes for your loved one's sudden change in behavior.

Common triggers:

- Physical discomfort—hunger, pain, temperature, fit of clothing

- Sounds—many people talking at once, loud music, constant beeping, or alarms

- Sights—bright lights

- Strong smells—perfume or smoke

- Tastes—bitter or acidic

Communication Using the Five Senses

Several scientific studies have noted how much of our communication is non-verbal. We rely heavily on body language and our senses to communicate with, to understand, and to respond to others. Non-verbal communication is just as important in dementia care, and there are several ways to have a meaningful engagement without using words. As the caregiver, frustration, confusion, and even guilt are all common emotions when you are at a loss to understand to what your loved one is trying to tell you. It is especially tiresome as you make multiple attempts to soothe them without much avail. Enhancing communication by engaging other senses gives you more tools to work with when your loved one is upset and you can't seem to figure out why. If a simple "Everything will be okay" doesn't work, then you can try rubbing their back or dimming the lights to calm them in other ways than verbal reassurance.

Touch

Tactile stimulation is brain stimulation because it is our brain that processes and recognizes the various textures, temperatures, and shapes that we are feeling. The Alzheimer's Association reports that encouraging tactile stimulation for those living with dementia and/or Alzheimer's disease increases both short-term and long-term memory, improves mood, and increases participation in daily activities.

Sensory boards are a popular tool used in long-term care settings because of the success they have in engaging someone living with dementia. A sensory board has a variety of objects with different textures and shapes. A sensory board is best for someone who uses their hands a lot, rummages through closets and drawers, or has a history of working with their hands.

Creating a Sensory Board

A sensory board is an easy and fun way to redirect your loved one. A sensory board has several different types of materials attached to an easy-to-hold-size board. The board can be as elaborate or as simple as you like, and you can use many household items that are already available to you. The items that you choose to place on the board should be a mixture of both familiar and new materials, so that your loved one can explore different sensations.

Items you will need:

- A sturdy, medium-sized piece of cardboard

- You can also use a sanded-down slab of wood

- Hot glue gun/glue

- A pair of scissors

- Ten to twenty tactile items like

- clothing

- sandpaper

- feathers

- yarn

- a belt buckle

- acorns

- fabric samples

- a piece of carpet

- a dried fruit pit

Directions:

- Collect the sensory items.

- Cut any large pieces into sample-sized squares.

- Lay out items on the cardboard.

- Hot glue items onto cardboard so that they are secure.

- For safety reasons, this step should only be done by the caregiver.

- Let dry.

- Hand the board to your loved one and run their hand over each piece.

Smell

Individuals living with dementia sometimes lose their ability to orient to person, place, or time. Aromatherapy is an effective way to momentarily reorient someone to the time and can be used in a variety of ways throughout the day.

Items you will need:

- A slow cooker

- Apples

Or

- An aromatherapy diffuser

- Essential oils

Aromatherapy to Orient to Time

Orientation to time means that the individual is aware of the time of the day, week, or year. They know (roughly) how old they are and what season it is.

A loss of orientation to time can cause an individual to put on layers of clothing during the summertime because they think it is winter, or can cause someone to skip meals because they believe they just ate when really, they haven't eaten anything since breakfast.

Baking cinnamon and apples a half hour or so before a meal is a gentle way to orient your loved one to know that it is almost time to eat and entice their appetite!

Aromatherapy to Ease Dementia Symptoms

Anxiety, fear, and depression can be common among individuals living with dementia. Incorporating essential oils into the care routine is a holistic way to reduce anxiety and will leave your home smelling amazing!

It is important to note that individuals may have sensitivity to certain smells, and, before the oils are diffused, make sure that your loved one will benefit from the aroma.

Common essential oils to reduce anxiety:

- Sweet Basil
- Lavender
- Lemon Balm
- Valerian

- Clary Sage

- Chamomile

- Jasmine

Common essential oils to reduce depression:

- Grapefruit

- Lavender

- Sandalwood

- Geranium

- Orange

- Rose

- Turmeric

Relaxation activities can offer respite on those high-intensity days. Dim the lights, run the diffuser with one of these calming scents, and play soothing soft music to calm both you and your loved one down in minutes!

Taste

Our taste buds change as we get older, and it is common to lose a bit of our sense of taste. To make dishes more enticing for your loved one, try adding a sweet touch. For example, instead of plain green beans, jazz them up with some butter and brown sugar. Not only are they more likely to eat them, but you've almost doubled the calorie intake they would have otherwise eaten.

Dietary restrictions often include low sodium and low sugar intake. In the nursing home, residents have the right to choose; if they are diabetic and want a piece of cake, we really can't stop them. However, if the diet is strict, check with your loved one's doctor to see if natural sugars are an appropriate alternative. Fruit smoothies and baked apples (with lots of butter) are sweet, flavorful, and can be offered throughout the day as snacks if food intake is low.

Hearing

Music is the number one tool I recommend when providing care. Music affects us deeply, and hearing a song we recognize provides a sense of self. Music has a beautiful way of moving past a diagnosis and will validate the memories and moments your loved one has experienced over the years.

Playing familiar songs that they can sing along to on the way to a doctor's appointment or social engagement will stimulate their mind in a way that prepares them for the engagement.

Create a special playlist with all your loved one's favorite songs, and listen to them together. If you don't know their favorite songs, here are a few patriotic songs and other popular sing-along songs that those in the Silent Generation demographic may enjoy:

- "Alexander's Ragtime Band" by Irving Berlin

- "America the Beautiful" by Ray Charles

- "Bicycle Built for Two" by Nat King Cole

- "For Me and My Gal" by Dean Martin

- "Give My Regards to Broadway" by Georg M. Cohan

- "Hail! Hail! The Gang's All Here" by D. A. Estrom

- "Home on the Range" by Frank Sinatra

- "I Love You Truly" by Al Bowlly

The songs of the Silent Generation might not work for the Baby Boomers, but creating a personalized playlist of songs you know your loved one will love is one of the best interventions you can provide.

Hearing loss can easily go undetected if your loved one has already received a dementia diagnosis because many of the signs and symptoms of hearing loss get mistaken for behaviors. Having regular checkups is an important aspect of care so that your loved one receives treatment for their sensory losses.

Sight

Your loved one may not always be able to tell you that their vision is worsening, and, if getting out to regular checkups is difficult, it is easy for vision loss to go unnoticed and even untreated. Vision loss is a more common occurrence as we age, and, like hearing loss, many of the symptoms of loss of sight get mistaken for dementia.

For instance, reduced depth perception and the ability to make out shapes and edges is a sign of vision loss, so you may notice your loved one is stepping over certain areas of the carpet or tile. This happens a lot when there are light and dark patterns in the flooring. The dark parts look like holes, and, as a precaution, they will step over them.

Using activities that rely heavily on the other senses, such as the sensory board and listening to music, will help engage your loved one in a way that won't strain their eyesight and will reduce any frustrations they may have as a result of not being able to see well.

Dementia care is a unique and sometimes challenging journey, and as a caregiver, you will find that many of the struggles and frustrations occur when you can't understand what it is they are trying to tell you. While their choice of words and sentence structure may be impaired, their ability to comprehend and respond appropriately to any given situation is not, and it is up to you to figure out what they are trying to tell you. Identifying patterns and taking note of any noticeable environmental factors, such as hunger, temperature, or loud noises, could help you hone in on what your loved one is responding to. If words are still just not enough, to communicate using all of your senses will allow you to convey your message or redirect them if they are feeling anxious.

Chapter Four

Approaches to Address Behaviors

I want to emphasize "getting to know them." Dementia is a group of symptoms, and those symptoms are unique to the individual. While most aspects of your loved one's personality will, of course, remain intact, you may find that there are significant characteristic or memory changes that, when you're faced with them as a caregiver, can be quite alarming!

In the context of caregiving, these changes in your loved one can make it feel as though you are caring for a stranger. For example, your mom suddenly begins to get angry and starts to yell at you for something you may or may not have done to her. Coming from a loved one, these high emotions can be hurtful and not easily shaken off. The behavior might stir up bad memories of being yelled at as a child, or, if you have always had a great relationship with her, the sudden anger directed at you can be taken quite personally.

No matter what your particular circumstances are, it becomes challenging to separate the person from the situation. Sure, your dad may have always had a smile on his face and a joke to tell, but that was before he depended on you to feed him. His sudden anger could be his way of asserting his independence in his care. This is where getting to know him is so important. Is his sudden burst of rage happening at a specific time of day or during a particular care task? It may seem sudden and unprovoked, but it may also be his way of communicating that he's not happy with the direction of this aspect of his care.

This chapter will go over the importance of maintaining your loved one's preferred routine, as well as highlight a few of the more common behaviors your loved one may demonstrate, such as forgetting who you are or asking to go home. By the end of the chapter, you will have approaches to identify dementia behaviors, and simple tools and interventions that you can use to redirect them so they feel more safe and secure in their environment.

Research and Understand Established Routines

It may be easier for you as a caregiver to keep your loved one on your schedule, but that doesn't mean it will work best for them. You may find their agitation increases as they are taken away from their normal routine. Routines and patterns are a caregiver's best friend, especially when caring for someone with Alzheimer's or other forms of dementia. Anger and agitation are sometimes caused by a change in routine, but can easily be dismissed as a symptom of dementia. This behavior might be a sign that your loved one is dissatisfied with the direction of their care. If you have had a close relationship with the person, you probably know to some extent what their normal routine has been. This information should be used to your benefit, so if they enjoy eating breakfast before they take their shower, for example, this preference should be honored. However, if you are not aware of these details, then striking a balance may take time, but that doesn't mean it can't be done.

For example, I once had a resident who, every day for fifty years, drank afternoon tea and watched her "shows" for an hour, then took a half-hour nap. But when she moved onto our unit, she became non-verbal. Without knowledge of this routine, we didn't know what was wrong with her. Since she always seemed to enjoy the morning activities, we naturally invited her to attend our afternoon socials. Although she accepted our invitation, she would quickly become agitated and would often try to get up from her wheelchair to walk back to her room. Since she so frequently tried to get up from her wheelchair, the nurses labeled her a fall risk, which meant that she couldn't go back to her room by herself for fear that she would fall. This made the situation worse, and, within a month, the afternoons had become almost intolerable for both her and the staff who were trying to soothe her. It wasn't until an old friend came to visit who happened to bring in her favorite tea and asked us to bring her a cup that we put two and two together!

The next day, we respected her routine, and there was never an incident like that again. Because we didn't know about this ritual, we forced her into a care plan that no doubt made her feel uncomfortable and one that took away her independence. Do that to anyone and you, too, will find that they "behave" in a negative way.

While not all situations will be so cut-and-dried, it will be necessary to investigate to understand. The first place to start when trying to establish a routine for your loved one is to get a notebook. Taking consistent and detailed notes of their behavior, response to care provisions, and other notable changes throughout the day will help you identify their preferences and efficiently manage a care practice that suits their preferred routine. The next section will discuss how to set up the notebook, and what information is essential for you to record.

Using a Notebook to Identify Patterns

Significant health changes rarely occur out of the blue, but because small or subtle symptoms can easily be explained away as part of the disease, notable declines or falls can seem sudden. Keeping a notebook and making daily entries is a beneficial tool when trying to identify patterns in behaviors, manage care tasks, and document incidents. In long-term care, we call this type of note-taking "documentation." Taking daily notes will help you notice more minor changes in their health and ability, which will better assist in you tracking the progress of their care.

Additionally, bringing your notebook to their doctor's appointments will help you reference changes or incidents accurately, so that the physician has full knowledge of what has happened since your loved one's last visit. To try and remember every aspect of your loved one's care can be exhausting, and you are more likely to forget the more pertinent details when trying to account for what happened.

Dementia can be an easy scapegoat when trying to explain a recent fall or change in behaviors, and I have heard of several patients whose care plan was changed after an incident because it was thought that dementia had caused it. For example, does their fall out of bed really make them a fall risk? Or was it simply because they got up in the middle of the night to go the bathroom and couldn't see? Distinguishing between the two can prevent prematurely transitioning your loved one to a walker or wheelchair when really the more reasonable solution is to buy a bedside commode and nightlight.

If you do not already keep notes, working this into your routine can be difficult. The best way to make journaling a habit is to write an entry at least once a day that reflects on any incidents or changes in behavior that occurred during the day, i.e., falls, loss of appetite, missed medications, sleeping throughout the day. Keep all your notes in one notebook or file to keep track of any changes in one easy-to-find place. To ensure that you can recall all the details of an incident, you should write down everything that happened as soon as you are able and try to avoid writing late at night or waiting until the next day, so you don't forget any important details. All entries should include the date and time of the incident.

Sample Entry:

Mom ate breakfast at eight. She ate all her eggs and one slice of toast. She spilled her orange juice but drank all her milk. After breakfast, I helped her change into her clothes. She could assist but struggled to keep her balance. Around two, I noticed that she was getting tired, and I asked her if she wanted to lie down, which she did and woke back up an hour later. When she woke up, we read together and sat outside and she enjoyed watching the birds. She ate dinner at five and ate 100 percent of her dinner.

Below are a few questions to get you started; they will only take a few minutes to answer.

1. What time(s) did they nap throughout the day?

2. How often and at what times did they need to go to the bathroom?

3. Did they raise their voice or start banging on the table or clapping their hands?

- If yes, at what time?

- What was their environment like at this time?

- Was there a lot of noise?

- Had you just gotten home?

- Was any care being provided?

- Was it too warm or too cold?

- Were all of the lights on?

4. At what time(s) did they seem most awake and engaged?

In addition to note-taking, keeping a section in your notebook that manages and tracks all their medication will be a helpful tool to take with you during their doctor's appointments. The next part will offer tips to keep track of all of their medicines and includes a sample chart to help you manage.

Medication Management

Medication management is a critical part of a caregiver's duty. A Medscape study found that 60 percent of older adults who manage their medication do so improperly, and 76 percent are more likely to experience a significant decline in their overall health than those who take all medicines as prescribed.[22]

As their caregiver, taking on medication management can be a daunting and time-consuming task because, let's be real, who really knows what the brown pill does versus what the little white one does?

Keeping the list of their medications in your notebook will mean that you have them on hand and can update the information as needed to ensure they will never miss a dose. Plus, it's an easy reference to take with you to all the doctor's appointments or to give to someone who will manage their medications in your stead.

To take on medication management, there are several key bits of information you will need to keep track of:

1. What is the name of the medication?

2. What does it look like?

3. What is the medication is used for?

4. At what time of day does it need to be taken?

5. Any special instructions, i.e., should this be taken with food?

6. What are possible side effects of the medication?

7. A place to sign off that the meds were taken for each day.

---

22 American Public Health Association, "Fact Sheet: Prescription Medication Use by Older Adults" MedScape, accessed April 1, 2019. https://www.medscape.com/viewarticle/501879.

Tip: Doctors talk fast, and it is hard to remember, once you leave, if they've prescribed a new medication or discontinued use of another. Take your journal with you to the doctor's appointment so you can quickly jot down everything they say!

MEDICATION NAME AND DESCRIPTION (COLOR/SIZE)	WHAT IS IT FOR?	WHAT TIME? (A.M./P.M.)	SPECIAL INSTRUCTIONS	SIDE EFFECTS	CHECK THAT YOU TOOK IT

Consistently taking notes on your loved one's routine will allow you to remember essential details more clearly, and you will be better able to identify subtle changes in their behavior or health. Take your notebook with you to every doctor's appointment so you can easily convey these changes to their doctor while in the office. It also is a helpful tool to manage all their medications, and if the doctor changes or adds a pill during their visit, you can update it right then and there. If you don't already journal, making documentation a part of your routine can be difficult at first, but if you are consistent and take notes every day, it will quickly become a habit that you'll find hard to break.

Common Behaviors

Two of the most common dementia behaviors I've heard family members express frustration over are when an individual doesn't recognize them and when an individual asks to go home (when they are already in their home). These behaviors can easily be explained away as a symptom of dementia. However, understanding these behaviors can open opportunities for caregivers to get to know their loved ones better during this new phase of their life and for you to explore and use different approaches to ensure they feel safe and secure in their environment.

What to Do When an Aging Parent Forgets Who You Are

A well-known and yet hurtful reality of Alzheimer's disease or other forms of dementia is the forgetfulness and memory loss that can occur. While the severity of memory loss varies in each case, many individuals in later stages of their diagnosis have been known to forget or not recognize important people in their life. Memory loss is particularly painful for family members to cope with when their parent or loved one misremembers who they are.

Forgetting the names of their children, forgetting that they have children, or mistaking their child for another person or family member is not uncommon for individuals living with Alzheimer's disease or other forms of dementia. And while this new reality may be shocking to the family member, to remind the patient that they've forgotten such an intimate detail about their own life can be quite upsetting to them.

When I worked in the nursing home, my training prepared me for these types of interactions. I would say hi to some residents who I'd been working with for years and knew that, while I might look familiar to them, they sometimes had no idea who I was. Although not being recognized did have an emotional impact on me, this is nothing compared to caregivers who are also daughters, sons, husbands, and wives. This is sometimes the most difficult thing for family members, and I want to offer tips on how to work through and cope with this specific aspect of dementia care.

Let Them Be Who They Are, No Questions Asked

Correcting and quizzing are two common responses to loss of recognition that I've witnessed both professional and family caregivers use over the years. At times, these types of approaches do work; however, in my experience, the intent of asking the question is to offer the caregiver reassurance or validation, rather than the person living with dementia or Alzheimer's.

The most common orientation questions are, "Mom, who am I?" "Who is this?" "Do you know where you are?" and "Do you know where you live?" The directness of the question can be confusing for someone living with dementia. Their memory recall is not as fast as ours, so undoubtedly, when faced with questions like these, the easiest answer is a sheepish laugh, followed by an "I don't know."

These types of questions also force the person to suddenly take back control of their situation and surroundings, which can be quite alarming. They've had to trust that the caregiver will provide for them, and it's our job to maintain that sense of safety at all times.

Understandably, these responses are coming from a place of being hurt, angry, or even fearful, because such blatant memory loss is a physical reminder of your loved one's diagnosis. However, there is an opportunity to reengage your loved one in a way that can help coax their memory. Being questioned can quickly shut them down. Instead, guide them and begin reminiscing, which is a beautiful and dignified way of prompting their remembrance.

We Remember Their Love When They Can No Longer Remember

Comprehending a life without memories is difficult. Memories mean so much to us. They provide us with a sense of self and stand as a reminder of the journey we have taken in this life. And the memories we share with the people closest to us become an intimate part of our identity. Alzheimer's may take these memories away from us, but the inability to remember does not have to redefine who we are, nor does it diminish the importance of the many moments that we have collected over the years.

Asking to Go Home

In care homes, shift changes are a particularly challenging time for residents, as they are watching staff putting on their coats to leave and talking about the things they have to do on their way home, like pick up the kids, make dinner, go shopping, etc. My shift ended well after the new shift started, and I would watch as the nurses and nurses' aides would struggle with the residents who wanted to go home too or who were concerned about their kids who would be stuck at school or at soccer practice. Obviously, their children were grown adults who had not had a soccer practice in many years, but, in that moment, as they processed the events happening around them, it became their reality.

To ask to go home can be confusing for family caregivers, particularly when their loved one is already at home. A notable number of individuals living with dementia will ask to go home. The question is often either their response to a feeling they have or a reaction to something someone else has said. It is a valid statement, even if they are sitting in their favorite chair in the place they have lived in for years.

When your loved one asks to go home, consider what else they may be trying to tell you.

Here are some questions you can ask yourself:

- What time of day is it when they ask to go home?

- Is it right before mealtime?

  - Maybe "home" means they are hungry, and they want to go home to make something to eat.

- Is it in the evening?

  - Call us creatures of habit, but when you spend a lifetime of leaving work at five to go home and make dinner, the routine can be hard to break. And why wouldn't it be? Don't activities like these give us a sense of purpose, sense of security, sense of self?

Whatever their reason for wanting to go home may be, reassuring them that they are already in their home will not always work. At this moment, it is imperative that we meet them in their reality. For any of the reasons listed above, your loved one wants to go home, and you should validate that feeling for them. Meeting them in their reality means that, even though you know they are in their home and are safe, you acknowledge that *they* don't feel this way at this time. To meet them in their reality, you should first identify what home means to them; for instance, are they referring to their childhood home? Or do they mean the home in which they raised their own family?

To do this, you can ask detailed questions like:

- What did your home look like?

- Did you have your own room, or did you have to share?

- Did you get along with your neighbors?

- What town did you live in?

Asking questions does two things: 1) it helps you decipher what past home they are referring to and 2) allows them to reminisce about the house they are missing. To tell them they are already at home will more than likely upset them, and if they are insistent on getting home, trying to reassure them that they don't have to go anywhere will make them feel trapped and confused. If they are adamant about leaving and continue to try to get out the door, try referencing the time and the weather to redirect them.

Sample Redirection Lines

If they are trying to leave, you can say, "It is freezing outside, and you don't have a coat. Why don't we have a cup of tea?"

If they have to go to pick up their kids from school, you can say, "Oh, it is only noon and school hasn't let out yet. That reminds me, I'm starting to get a little hungry; why don't we get some lunch?"

If they have to go home to make dinner or their spouse will wonder where they are, you can say, "What was [spouse's name]'s favorite meal? Did you enjoy cooking dinner? Why don't we go get a snack, and you can teach me how to make [the dish]?"

All of these statements validate their reference to home and aim to redirect them to another activity. Redirection won't work every time, but you will find that certain activities will work better than others. Food always seemed to be a great redirection tool for the residents, and if you sit with them and share a cup of tea or a snack, by the end, they've forgotten their desire to go home.

> **Exercise:** Write down the days and times when they ask to go home and a brief description of the circumstances, and reflect on your entries at the end of the month. With a bit of understanding, you will be better prepared to address their desire to go home.

_____

_____

_____

_____

_____

_____

_____

_____

_____

_____

Approaches to Behaviors

Professional caregivers have developed several approaches to addressing a variety of behaviors that stem from a dementia diagnosis. Addressing behaviors in a way that ensures your loved one feels heard and validated is essential. Not only are you upholding their dignity, but individuals with dementia still know when they are not being taken seriously. To address behaviors abrasively can be upsetting, and can cause needless stress and confusion for them. In this section, you will learn how to deal with behaviors while in public, how to use validation therapy, redirection, and the benefits of staying in their reality.

Five Ways to Defuse Dementia Triggers While Out in Public

A noisy and crowded space is an overwhelming environment to be in and will easily trigger anxiety or irritability for someone living with dementia. This makes places like a doctor's waiting room or a crowded restaurant hot spots for dementia behavior flare-ups. Removing them from the environment may not always be an option, so finding ways to keep their focus on you is important.

The stimulus from everything happening around them makes it hard for them to focus on any one thing, but this is what they need to do so that they can feel safe and in control.

1. Make Physical Contact

The sensation of you holding their hand or patting their back anchors them to you. You've created a foundation that they can focus their attention on.

2. Maintain Eye Contact

Seeing a familiar face is a good reminder that they are not alone. Even if they can't quite remember who you are, they know that you are with them, and that will calm their fears of being lost.

3. Communicate

Engaging them in conversation is an easy distraction from everything else that is going on around them. Keeping it light and on a topic that they can easily engage in is important so that they don't become flustered over their own words.

If conversations aren't possible, start singing a song you know they love. Understandably, you are in public and don't want everyone to hear you, but putting modesty aside to prevent an episode is sometimes worth the public serenade. Plus, more than likely, your loved one will have no problem singing right along with you.

4. Relax

Whether consciously or not, your loved one is looking to you to gauge the safety of the environment around them. If you are flustered, they will pick up on this emotion and become flustered, too. No matter how hectic the situation you may find yourself in, take a step back to breathe, re-center, and smile. Your loved one will mimic you and begin calming down, too.

5. Create a Moment of Calm

The best way to unwind from a chaotic day out is to come home, dim the lights, and put on soft music. Dimmed lights is the best thing I have found to calm a situation because bright lights can be a trigger for individuals living with dementia. To dim the lights tells the body it is time to relax, and is also helpful to prompt an afternoon nap.

Adequately addressing dementia behaviors in public is difficult. Many people in this situation search for the quickest way to calm their loved one down. But often a rapid response from the caregiver and frantic attempts to quell the situation only make things worse. To slow down and assess the situation offers you an opportunity to connect with them and to address their feelings rather than the behaviors, which will provide much better results.

Validation Therapy

Validation therapy was created by Naomi Feil. Validation therapy is a non-medical intervention technique that seeks to meet the person living with dementia where they are by acknowledging the emotions they are feeling, rather than the actions or behaviors that they are demonstrating.

Receiving validation from others, no matter the form, can have a powerful effect on all of us. Validation lets us know we've been heard and that our feelings are important. Both giving and receiving validation can provide our interactions with a strong foundation for communication and a better opportunity for a peaceful resolution. Validation transcends the need for spoken dialogue and targets the human need to have our emotions heard.

Validation is a great communication technique and a crucial tool to use with your loved one living with dementia or Alzheimer's. Their speech may be impaired, but that does not mean they stop communicating with us in other ways. And when we use validation, we first try our very best to focus on the emotion they are feeling in that moment and not on the words they are trying to use. Below is a list of some ways to provide validation to a loved one in your care:

1. Listen to the Tone of Their Voice

At first, identifying their exact emotion may be difficult, so a good starting point may be to narrow it down to a few emotions. Are they sad, anxious, or afraid? Or are they happy, excited, or playful?

To do this, we may need to ask a few questions or engage in a bit more conversation. You can say, "I can see you are upset, can I help?" This conveys that we recognize something is wrong and that we are there for them.

We should then give them an opportunity to express themselves, even if the words they use don't make sense to us. As they finish, we can validate their feelings by saying, "You have every right to be upset," or "I can see how that can be upsetting." And, if it feels appropriate to redirect the conversation, "How about we go for a walk and get something to drink? I think you deserve to relax for a bit."

2. Mirror Your Facial Expression to Theirs

A furrowed brow or a worried look can say a thousand words. You may not know what they are worried about, but you can see that they are obviously upset.

In these moments, you should mirror their expression. If they have a furrowed brow, so should you. If they are smiling, we smile right back! Mirroring their facial expression sends an unspoken validation that you understand how they are feeling.

3. The Importance of Touch

A part of validation therapy is being engaged. If they are pacing back and forth or if they have their hands clenched together, there may be something wrong. Try rubbing their back or holding their hand as they are speaking to you. Walk with them if they are pacing, and listen as they vent their feelings. If it seems appropriate, try finding chairs. If you sit down, they will most likely sit with you, which gives them a rest from all the pacing.

It can be extremely frustrating to watch as your loved one struggles to communicate, but you should always allow them to try. They still have feelings that are worth listening to, and this technique allows our loved ones to know that they've been heard and understood.

Stay in Their Reality

Individuals living with dementia or Alzheimer's will often speak of their younger years as if it were their current reality. They tell stories of their childhood home, their parents, and will even feel the need to go home and make dinner for their young children. Sometimes the need for this reality is so great that they become anxious and even angry when they can't find what, in their mind, should be there.

How trapped and powerless they must feel in these moments! Imagine if we woke up one day and everyone we knew and loved was no longer there, or if our once routine and purposeful lives were now only a distant memory.

As a caregiver, you've most likely had to "fib" at one time or another. When asked where their mother or father was, you may have said they were at the store; when asked if they could go home, you may have said it was too cold to go outside; or, when asked when their kids would be there, you may have replied that they were at school that day. These types of answers may not always work as well as you hope they do, but they can offer your loved one comfort and peace of mind in knowing that their mother is still alive and will soon return.

I've had many people ask about the ethical implications of lying to someone with dementia or Alzheimer's. However, there are multiple benefits from the practice of being in their reality for both them and you. When you engage them in their stories of the past, you learn and connect on their terms, not yours. However, the question of whether we should lie to individuals with dementia comes up a lot in the aging field, and, as a result, many caregivers choose to use the practice of reality orientation.

Reality orientation is the method of reminding the person with dementia or Alzheimer's of the facts of their current situation. If they wonder where their parents are, we tell them that their parents are no longer living, or that they can't go home because they no longer live in their childhood home. We will also remind them of the actual date and time, and their current living situation.

In my experience, reality orientation causes anxiety and can even scare the person with dementia or Alzheimer's. Arguing with someone who has dementia is futile and will often exacerbate the situation. Whether we think they are making up these stories or not, when we attempt to correct them, we are essentially calling them a liar and taking away any sense of control they may get from telling these stories.

If you feel more comfortable with reality orientation, you should always use it in the gentlest possible manner, so as to not embarrass or shame the individual who has forgotten. The Alzheimer's Association also stresses the importance of communication with those living with dementia and Alzheimer's and notes that communication requires patience, understanding, and good listening skills.

Reminisce

Reminiscing with friends and family that we have spent meaningful moments with throughout our lives is a fun and engaging pastime that many of us have taken part in at some point. Remembering the good times or the simpler times offers all of us a chance to reflect on all that has happened in our lives so far, and an opportunity to take note of the growth we've achieved over the years. It is a compassionate activity and reassures us that, while we may have changed, many of us are still grounded in the roots laid down during these special moments.

For an individual living with dementia, short-term memory loss is a common symptom of the diagnosis and creating new memories may be difficult. Short-term memory loss is quite upsetting for those who interact with the person daily, because the conversation you had only moments ago seems to have disappeared entirely from your loved one's memory. As mentioned earlier, it is quite common to want to question or prompt your loved one during these moments, which can be upsetting for them when they realize they've forgotten so much. Instead, if you work to their strengths and engage their long-term memory, you will find that your loved one remembers so much of their life and is able to laugh and reminisce with you over shared memories, and even tell you stories that you may never have heard before.

Depending on their state of mind at the time, a reminiscing activity may start slowly, but once they warm up and realize how familiar these stories are to them, they will become more easily engaged. Asking broader questions is a great way to start the reminiscing process because it allows them time to fill in gaps in their memory. For instance, asking "What was your maid of honor's name?" is too specific, and immediately forces them to recall a detail, which switches the focus from reminiscing to memory recall. Instead, ask "Did you have a bridal party?" This kind of question asks them for a simple yes or no answer and allows them the freedom to elaborate on the memory, if it is one that is easy for them to recall. If they say no, you can ask another, even broader question, like "Did you enjoy planning your wedding?" Through conversation and dialogue, you will find that your loved one begins to remember so much more.

Here are a few topics for conversation starters:

- Childhood home

- Siblings

- Childhood friends/school/neighborhood

- Childhood games (i.e., jump-rope, hopscotch, kickball)

- Nicknames

- Parents/grandparents

- Special occasions (prom, graduation, wedding day)

- Career(s)

- Traditions

- Owning a home

Many people living with dementia related to Alzheimer's remember their childhood through their young adult life quite vividly. Looking at old photos or discussing old family recipes or family vacations will prompt and orient their memory, so they are ready to answer your reminiscing questions.

There are a variety of approaches you can use to address dementia behaviors. Before any intervention, you should try to understand the cause of the behavior so that you can help your loved one avoid situations/environments that they find upsetting or stressful. To better understand how your loved one is reacting to their environment, you should document daily the various aspects of their day and care routine. Daily documentation will allow you to better understand subtle changes in their health and disease progression that may otherwise go unnoticed, and becomes a helpful tool when trying to describe to their physician an incident that occurred in the recent past.

To forget or not recognize important people in their life, and a frequent request to go home, are both common behaviors of individuals with dementia. These behaviors are confusing and can be the most difficult for family caregivers to understand. To understand these behaviors makes it easier to cope with otherwise significant reminders of your loved one's disease progression. There are several interventions you can use to redirect and interact with your loved one so that they can successfully interact and even remember important moments in their life. Incorporating these approaches into your care routine allows you to engage in meaningful moments together.

Chapter Five

Activities to Ease Care Tasks

Activities of daily living, doctor's appointments, and medication management are parts of a treatment plan that aims to keep an individual physically healthy. As you know, the person you are caring for is more than a medical diagnosis, so a constant focus on this aspect of their lives can distort their sense of self and hurt their emotional well-being. Incorporating non-medical activities into the care plan allows your loved one to concentrate on him/herself. Activities that you are both engaged in will not only be fun, but also strengthen the bond between you, which in turn eases some of the stresses of the caregiving experience.

As an activity professional, I saw firsthand the power activities can have for an individual in a care center. Recreational pursuits allow us to remember and embrace aspects of ourselves that are not defined by or dependent on good health. I don't mean activities like bingo or group birthday parties. These are too generic and work only to pass the time. The moments in which I saw the most benefit by far involved smaller and more natural activities, like baking chocolate chip cookies together in the kitchen or having a conversation about things like when they bought their first car or how they met their spouse.

Without medical tools at my disposal, I had to find holistic ways to intervene and calm a resident who had become anxious or angry. Certain activities, like listening to music or bringing up a fond memory, became great ways to redirect and reengage a resident if they were feeling anxious or fearful. Over time, I knew exactly how to "treat" each resident if they started to demonstrate a particular dementia symptom. In this framework, activities aren't just used to pass the time or to have fun. These interactions are tools crafted to ensure that your loved one can thrive throughout their day.

Why did these interactions work? Because I was with them at that moment. I was listening to what they were saying to me, even if I didn't understand their words. I knew that they weren't just behaving in a particular way because they had dementia, but instead were trying to communicate with me in a new way. I gave them the time and space to engage with me, which ensured that their autonomy in the activity remained intact. It is easy to want to rush through caregiving tasks, especially when you are overwhelmed with all that you have to do, but rushing through offers no time for your loved one to process or communicate to you what they would like or need to be done.

As you provide care to an older adult, it is crucial that they remain engaged in the process, particularly individuals living with Alzheimer's disease or other forms of dementia. Just because someone can no longer take care of themselves does not mean that they give up their rights to being human. As their caregiver, it is important that, in addition to providing for their physical care, you are continuing to uphold their dignity and their autonomy.

In private caregiving moments, individuals in need of care will do anything to maintain control and dignity in the situation. Sometimes this even means that they will yell and could also become aggressive. These are your signs to step back and reevaluate. You may need to get this task done as quickly as possible, but they are telling you they are uncomfortable and you need to find out why. It could just be because you are moving too fast for them, and all you need to do is adjust your pace. Maybe the whole experience is overwhelming. Try adding soft sing-along music while doing the task. With this subtle distraction, your loved one will focus their attention on singing the song rather than yelling at you for doing something wrong.

I have found that dementia can make the person extremely sensitive to their caregiver's emotions and they will quickly pick up on how you are feeling. If they sense that you are disengaged in the process or rushing through a care task, they will more than likely become anxious and angry themselves.

Activities serve as preparation for caregiving tasks. Establishing a routine is one of the best things you can do as a family caregiver. Including activities that are designed to engage and assist in the caregiving process into your routine is just as important because, when done right, they will help your loved one's fine motor skills, speech, memory, and mood. We do this all the time in our day-to-day routine, like stretching before a run or practicing a speech before a big presentation.

This chapter offers tips on how you can establish routines. It focuses on activities that will exercise their body and mind, which in turn makes care tasks easier for them.

Establishing a Morning Routine

The start of a new day opens so many opportunities, and how we approach each morning will set the tone of your loved one's mood and behaviors for the rest of the day. They are not going to be able to go at the same pace as you, even if you need them to. Offering space and time for them to wake up and to process the steps you need them to complete is critical to their ability to assist you in the care process and maintain as much independence as they can.

For example, when picking out an outfit in the morning, it may be easy to pick out the first sweater you see in their closet, but when you offer them a choice between the blue shirt and the green sweater, you are engaging them in the process and encouraging them to make their own decisions. In doing so, you've helped them start the morning with a self-esteem boost and allowed them to maintain their autonomy. Limiting the number of choices you offer to two or three won't overwhelm them and will enable them to point or gesture if they are non-verbal.

A routine helps all of us get through each day; however, from time to time, something in our system no longer works, and we have to change it so that we can stay on pace for the rest of the day. The same goes for the routine you and your loved one have established; as their caregiver, be mindful of sudden changes in mood or response to daily tasks. For example, Mom may start yelling at breakfast. This only happens on Mondays and Wednesdays, which happen to be the same days she has a shower right before breakfast. The negative feelings she has toward her shower are carrying over into the rest of the day. In this case, there are a couple of things you can try: 1) Offer more time between shower and breakfast, so that she can calm down. Maybe even play some of her favorite music in her room to relax, too. 2) Change the time of her shower to after breakfast. 3) Assess whether a shower is still an appropriate method of care.

Beneficial Activities in the Morning

By starting each day with a morning stretch followed by a trivia or reminiscing session, you empower your loved one to keep the body and mind active. This order is important. We can think of stretching as a warm-up session for the mind. In the morning stretch, your loved one will begin to focus on following your movements. This time gives them an opportunity to become acquainted with the other people or noises in the room. Once they have had that time to focus and orient, they will be ready for trivia. Trivia promotes memory recall and encourages them to think quickly.

Morning Stretches

Waking up to morning stretches is a great way to get the body prepared for the day. It can be before or after the care routine.

Leg stretches

- While sitting, stick legs straight out in front and hold for ten seconds, then release.

- While sitting with both legs straight out, alternate toe taps on the floor.

- While sitting, put the right leg out and point the toe; then left leg out and point the toe.

- March to the tune of "When the Saints go Marching In" (and have them sing along).

Arm stretches

- Reach both hands above your head and bring them back down to your side.

- Pretend to row to the tune of "Row, Row, Row Your Boat" (and have them sing along).

- Reach your right arm up, bend your elbow, and pat yourself on the back. Repeat on the left.

- Bring your right arm over your chest and hold your elbow with your left hand. Repeat on the left.

Upper body

- Shrug your shoulders up and down.

- Roll your shoulders backward.

- Roll your shoulders forward.

- Bring your right shoulder up to the ear and hold it. Repeat on left.

Head and neck

- Gently look to the left.

- Gently look to the right.

- Gently look up to the sky.

- Gently look down to the floor.

Trivia for Memory Recall

Trivia should be offered after the morning exercise because it gives your loved one a chance to warm up their mind. The more they get right, the more confident they will be throughout the rest of their day.

Idioms:

- It is raining (cats and dogs)
- A penny for (your thoughts)
- A bird in the hand is worth (two in the bush)
- A blessing (in disguise)
- A chip on (your shoulder)
- A dime (a dozen)
- A Doubting (Thomas)
- A drop in (the bucket)
- A fool and his money are easily (parted)
- A house divided against itself (cannot stand)
- A leopard can't change his (spots)
- A penny saved is (a penny earned)
- A picture paints (a thousand words)
- A piece (of cake)
- A slap on (the wrist)
- A taste of your (own medicine)
- Let sleeping dogs (lie)
- Let the cat out of (the bag)
- It takes two to (tango)

- Don't cry over (spilled milk)

Famous Pairs:

- Adam and (Eve)

- Bert and (Ernie)

- Fred and (Ginger)

- Batman and (Robin)

- Bonnie and (Clyde)

- Simon and (Garfunkel)

- Lucy and (Ethel) / (Ricky)

- Butch Cassidy and (the Sundance Kid)

- Dr. Jekyll and (Mr. Hyde)

- Sherlock Holmes and (Dr. Watson)

- Peanut butter (and jelly)

- Gilligan and (the Skipper)

- Tom Sawyer and (Huckleberry Finn)

- Tom and (Jerry)

- Abbott and (Costello)

- Morecombe and (Wise)

- Scooby-Doo and (Shaggy)

- Macaroni and (Cheese)

- Chip and (Dale)

- Calvin and (Hobbes)

In just two activities, you have allowed them to orient naturally to their surroundings and to stimulate their mind and body so that they are awake and ready to take on the day. By this time, you are ready for breakfast, so transitioning your trivia session into a conversation on favorite foods or reminiscing about old family recipes will cue them that it is time to eat, even if their body is not telling them they are hungry.

Mealtime Activities to Entice an Appetite

Food is an essential part of the human experience. While, of course, it is necessary for our survival, mealtimes and food choices have defined cultures around the world and stand as an indispensable social tradition. Whether we know how to cook or not, as individuals, we often get to choose what we want and don't want to eat. We all have that one favorite go-to meal or indulge in comfort foods when we are feeling down. The autonomy in food choice is often overlooked, and the way food shapes our day-to-day routine could go unappreciated until it is gone.

Buying and preparing food can become more difficult as we get older, for many different reasons. For those who are no longer able or willing to drive, a trip to the grocery store means relying on public transportation or asking a friend or family member to take them. Or, if they are willing, carrying in grocery bags or putting food away on top shelves can start to become cumbersome. For those with memory impairments, leaving the stove on or overcooking food becomes a serious safety concern. And for those who had little to no culinary expertise, cooking a well-balanced meal becomes less and less of a priority. This decline in ability, however, does not mean that the social and cultural significance of meal prep and food choice goes away.

I once worked with a resident who would become emotional very quickly, and I would try everything to comfort her: playing soft music, sitting with her and holding her hand, and reading aloud, all in an attempt to soothe her. It wasn't until a cold fall day, when we decided to make chicken noodle soup for our afternoon activity, that I realized that all that this woman needed was a hot bowl of homemade soup. She smiled through the entire prep stage, and, after taking her first bite, she sighed so loudly and exclaimed, "This reminds me of my mother!" From then on, we made sure she got a bowl of soup with every meal, and, while it didn't always do the trick, we at least knew that she was eating something that brought her comfort and something she would have chosen if she was still able to prepare her own meals.

For some, the times we eat become the foundation for the day ahead, like my grandfather, "Pop," who every morning would wake up early, go to WaWa for a paper and coffee, and then come back to sit at the head of the table and eat a bowl of cereal—most of the time, out of an old Cool Whip container. These steps were a major part of his routine that happened every morning for at least the twenty-plus years I knew him. When he wasn't sitting at the table in the morning, we immediately noticed the change, and questioned it. This routine made up a part of who he was, and, if he were no longer able to do this on his own, it was a routine that I think everyone in the family knew should not be broken.

As a family caregiver, ensuring your loved one not only eats, but eats a healthy and well-balanced meal, is a challenge. Many older adults in need of assistance in food preparation and feeding will lose their choice in meal preference because it is easier for the caregiver to serve the same dish for everyone. While, of course, this is entirely understandable, if the caregiver does not already have a healthy lifestyle, the older adult in their care will most likely take on these eating habits, which can have severe effects on their health.

In addition to unhealthy food choices, loss of appetite and difficulty chewing or swallowing food are two major barriers for older adults to maintaining a healthy diet. Weight loss and weight gain become common and harmful symptoms, especially for those living with dementia and Alzheimer's. Ensuring your loved ones maintain the proper intake of calories in a day becomes a top priority in maintaining their physical well-being.

Here are some activity ideas to make mealtimes more enticing for you and your loved one:

1. Talk about Food

Start talking about food a half-hour or so before an actual meal. You can ask them how they would make their favorite recipe or discuss the menu for an upcoming celebration meal. Talking about food becomes a cue for them to orient themselves to hunger. Especially for those who are not oriented to time, they may not realize that it is a "normal" time to eat.

2. Make a Home-Cooked Meal

Preparing a meal at home is a fun and engaging activity that leaves the entire house smelling delicious. The smell of dinner cooking is a great way to stimulate your loved one's appetite and is another great way to help orient them to mealtime. If you know ahead of time what is on the menu, discuss the recipe with your loved one throughout the day. It gives them something to look forward to, and they will be more interested in eating the meal.

3. Pick Out the Recipes Together

If they are willing and able to help, go through old family recipes together or scope out new ones online or in a magazine. Once the recipe is picked out, go to the store together to pick up the ingredients. They can smell the fresh produce as you put it in the cart and help you by listing off the rest of the items on the list. When we allow them to have a say in the menu plan, there is a greater chance they will enjoy the meal, as it promotes their independence and autonomy.

4. Cook Together

Baking and cooking activities can be a ton of fun, but they also require the use and practice of motor skills. Have them assist in mixing in the ingredients or stirring them all together. These steps require minimal assistance while still being essential to the process. Cooking activities were by far the most popular with the residents; cooking is fun and familiar, and it offers a wonderful sense of accomplishment to see a meal through until the end.

5. Eat Together

Eating is a social activity, and your loved one is much more likely to eat if someone is sitting there eating and talking with them. Try discussing some favorite meals you had as a child, or other priceless memories that occurred around the dinner table. Even if you provide them with assistance in feeding, to sit down with them and eat at the same time cues them to eat and helps dignify the experience.

Music and Memory

Music is a truly magical tool in memory care and should be utilized in all aspects of the care routine. I have watched as individuals who haven't spoken in years belted out the lyrics to their favorite song, and someone who barely had the strength to open their eyes started tapping their toes when a good melody came on the radio. The songs of our past are so deeply rooted into us that they are often the last thing to go through a cognitive decline process. Music offers an anchor to their selves that, without the caregiver's intervention in maintaining the connection, would otherwise be lost. This is why it is so essential that music is incorporated into your care routine.

There are several different ways of listening to music that will help ease the care routine so that your loved one is relaxed throughout the process. Depending on the scenario, a variety of types of music should be gathered and used as tools to support you throughout the day. For instance, in the morning as you start the day, playing songs whose lyrics they can quickly recall, like their favorite songs or familiar sing-along songs, will prompt them to focus their mind on the tasks ahead of them. Once they gain confidence in remembering the song, they are more willing and able to focus their mind on the care tasks and will be better able to assist you in the process. Or, if you are looking for a quieter afternoon after a busy morning out running errands, playing relaxing music will set the mood for them to quietly listen to the soothing melody.

Music can also help intervene with dementia symptoms such as anger or anxiety. If your loved one is spiritual, singing hymns or gospel songs like "Yes, Jesus Loves Me" or "He's Got the Whole World in His Hands" can help comfort them in times of distress. Hold their hand and gently try to console them while you sing to them to create a safe space. To engage with them while they are listening to music helps remind them of their spiritual connection in a more profound way than watching a sermon on TV could.

Or, if your loved one is in a particularly good mood, putting on songs that they can dance to is a great way to get their body moving in a more natural and fun direction than an exercise routine could. Don't be afraid to dance or sing along to the songs with them because, when you engage with them, you create moments that you get to keep with you, and through music, you will find that your loved one is still very much alive inside, even if they are no longer able to communicate with you. There is a documentary on this subject that I've watched too many times to count because of how powerful its message is! *Alive Inside: A Story of Music and Memory* was released in 2014 by Dan Cohen and portrays the power music has on individuals living with dementia.[23]

Engaging in activities with your loved one with dementia eases the care tasks because it elicits meaningful participation from them in a way that they can process and understand. Activities offer step-by-step instructions that, when done during or before a care activity, prepare an individual with dementia to orient to the task. Because of busy schedules, it is easy to rush through specific care tasks, especially once you've done them for some time and they have become a bit routine. Establishing a morning routine offers an opportunity to slow it down and to engage your loved one's strengths or exercise the body and mind so that they can maintain their health and independence for as long as possible. Incorporating activities like listening to music during difficult care tasks, such as showering or mealtime, gives your loved one a definite point of focus to distract them from any anxiety they may have during care provision. Including activities in your care routine may seem like an added step; however, in doing so, you provide your loved one with an opportunity to participate in their care, which in turn helps you provide care with ease.

23 *Alive Inside: A Story of Music and Memory*, directed by Michael Rossato-Bennett, (Projector Media and the Shelley & Donald Rubin Foundation, 2014), DVD. http://www. aliveinside.us/.

Part Two

Part Two

Release Guilt—
Explore Care Options

Chapter Six
Managing Difficult Aspects of Care

It can be hard to separate the caregiving tasks from the person you are providing care to. After a while, activities of daily living become routine and the process can become a bit second nature, which helps you get the job done but can also cause you to move too quickly while you provide care. A separation between the tasks and person reduces the quality of care you are able to provide because you lose sight of the care recipient's preference and even response. Such oversight is quite common in long-term care facilities, and, as a result, many in the senior living industry have pushed nursing homes to adopt a culture change toward more mindful care provision.

In this chapter, we will discuss the origins of person-centered care and how its use can help you manage difficult aspects of care. Assisting someone else with their activities of daily living requires a focus on the person's preference and an understanding that, while someone needs assistance, they still deserve to be active participants, rather than passive recipients, in the care they receive. Family caregivers have a much better chance of offering effective person-centered care because they are providing care to a limited number of people. Certain aspects of care can be more difficult than others, and the following sections will focus on the impact falls, urinary tract infections (UTIs), and memory loss can have on both the care recipient and the caregiver.

Incorporating Person-Centered Care

Since 1987, when the Pioneer Network announced their initiative on culture change, nursing homes have promoted the concept of person-centered care. This culture change bases its concept of senior care on the idea that caregiving should not use a one-size-fits-all approach and that we must provide care in a way that respects a person's individuality and promotes both dignity and respect.[24] Incorporating the concept has proven difficult because caregiving is made up of concrete tasks like brushing your teeth or assistance in feeding, which make focusing on the individual's preference somewhat obscure. Family caregivers are much more likely to successfully provide person-centered care because they know the person they are caring for and are limited to providing care to only one or two people at a time.

Culture change is more philosophical in practice and depends on the caregiver making a conscious decision to uphold the care recipient's preference throughout the caregiving process. For instance, if your mom has always been a bit modest and prefers to take a shower as soon as she wakes up in the morning, she would most likely prefer to maintain her early morning schedule and would need you to be sensitive to her being uncomfortable with having someone else bathe her. This also means you have to plan in advance for an extra amount of time to meet her needs and still make it to work on time.

This understanding requires a care-preference conversation, which can be difficult to have if neither one of you has considered this aspect. Every family operates on a different level of ability when it comes to communication, so, if this is something you

---

24   The Pioneer Network, last modified 2019. https://www.pioneernetwork.net/.

have struggled with in the past, it may be helpful to bring a set of predetermined questions with you to the conversation. While you are there to discuss your loved one's preference, that doesn't mean that your capability and preference should be left out of the conversation. Bring your time schedule and time constraints, as well as a list of the care tasks you are uncomfortable with, so you can bring them up at the meeting.

I've known care recipients to push back or break down during this type of conversation because, despite the fact that you are trying to help them maintain their independence, it is still a sensitive topic. If you find that they feel uncomfortable or become defensive, try to remember that they are discussing (for example) the fact that they are no longer able to go to the bathroom on their own. These are intimate details that even families or close loved ones don't always share with one another. Patience and understanding are needed to make them comfortable and trusting that you have nothing but their best interest at heart.

For caregivers of someone living with Alzheimer's disease or other forms of dementia, a care conversation may not be possible; however, there are a number of ways you can maintain their independence and sense of control while you provide care. Here are a few examples of details of care that maintain control and independence.

Assistance in feeding:

- Give them options at mealtime

- Tell them what is on their plate

- Tell them what food they are about to take a bite of

- Provide a sip of water or juice between each new food

- Change their clothes if they get food on them

- Wipe their mouth when they are done

- Talk to them during the meal

- Eat with them

Assistance in going to the bathroom:

- Try to use briefs only as a backup

- Take them to the bathroom when they ask

- Don't ask them in public or loudly if they have to go to the bathroom

Assistance in walking:

- Walk with them daily, with or without their walker

- Offer physical therapy if available

- Do leg exercises with them daily

- Offer them encouragement to move around

Mindful caregiving is a practice that refocuses caregiving on the person. To manage your loved one's care requires a certain degree of patience and understanding, particularly as their disease progresses. Sometimes even seasoned family caregivers are faced with symptoms or situations that cause them to reconsider their ability to provide care. Medication side effects, falls, UTIs, and memory loss are four of the most common, because they can be so unpredictable and because of their effects on the health and well-being of an older adult. Maintaining a mindful caregiving practice through these times can prove difficult, but there are certain ways to manage your loved one's care that uphold both their dignity and your sanity.

Time Management

Providing care to a family member or loved one can quickly
consume your day. The once quasi-part-time care you offered
before becomes a full-time gig. When you are in the thick of it,
additional tasks easily go unnoticed; however, that doesn't mean
you won't feel it beginning to seep into other aspects of your life.
Without compensating for the additional time you've assigned to
your caregiver to-do list, your loved one's progressive care needs
could cause you stress, exhaustion, and even burnout.

Identifying as the primary caregiver means you have assumed
the role of manager of their care. Any good manager knows that
they need to have clear communication, the ability to delegate,
and a supportive team to succeed. To say that family caregiving is
just what you do is an understatement. There are real emotions
involved here, and conversations and planning are so essential
to ensure that everyone involved in the process is on board or, at
the very least, understands why certain decisions must be made.

It is understandable to want to do everything yourself, to
believe that you can do it all, but is that fair to you? This is
where delegating becomes key. It is critical to understand that,
even though you were able to step up and provide care when
your parents or loved one needed you, that does not mean that
everyone else in your life will feel able to do this, or will even
know how to.

For instance, your sister may live too far away to take your mom
to her doctor's appointments every Thursday, but, since she
is concerned for your mom's care, she calls you every week to
remind you of the appointment. Infuriating, right? Of course
you remember, because it was you who scheduled the weekly

appointment in the first place! However, there is an opportunity here to engage your sister in the care process in a more useful and less frustrating way. Ask her to make a monthly calendar of all of your mom's appointments, a list of the physicians' names, and the contact information for each. Engaging her in the care process by giving her a job that helps you still validates her concern for your mom's care and intervenes before she can come up with another way of becoming involved that is less productive.

Knowing your own strengths as a caregiver is a great place to start when you are trying to find ways to delegate your responsibilities. Would the meal prep and assistance in feeding be easier to manage if you didn't also have to go grocery shopping? Ask that friend who is always asking how they can help you to pick up a few things for you the next time they go to the store.

Do you struggle with handling certain dementia behaviors that result from specific care tasks, like assisting your loved one in taking a shower or getting dressed? Consider hiring a part-time care assistant who is trained and, quite frankly, is used to being yelled at for these types of caregiving acts. In the next chapter, we will go over how to have a conversation about care, but, to have that conversation, you must be prepared and know what you are comfortable with and what makes you uncomfortable within the caregiving process.

It is okay to say that you don't want to be responsible for a particular aspect of your loved one's care; it is knowing this ahead of time and being able to communicate it to them that is key. Knowing your limits will help guide the conversation so you can identify what can be done by you and what will need to be outsourced to others.

Ask your care support team to identify their preferences in providing care as well. Your brother may be very comfortable with taking your mom to all of her doctor's appointments but have no desire to help make dinner for her every night. Knowing this as you make your care plan will make your job a whole lot easier. As you put your plan into action, remember to check in with your family members to see if the situation continues to work for them. There are plenty of jobs to do, and, if you or they find that something isn't working out, it is better to know this right away than run the risk of frustration or burnout.

Just like a manager, as the primary caregiver, you will have to make a lot of unilateral (and sometimes unpopular) decisions. In my experience, discord between family members often occurs when the primary caregiver determines something without discussing it with the others in the support team first. They may not understand all of your choices, but, if you engage them in the care process and explain that your loved one's comfort and safety is your priority, you validate their concerns and make space for them to join you in the decision-making process.

Falls and Safety Concerns

It is hard not to talk about falls and other safety concerns when we discuss the care of an older adult. The industry has focused so much time and resources on fall prevention, yet falls still happen. It is important here to distinguish between increased mobility and fall prevention when we talk about falls. Too often, we choose to keep an individual immobile for fear that they will fall and break a hip. While this is a very serious concern, the limitations put upon people who have spent their whole lives being mobile can be extremely difficult for them to get used to and to maintain.

Frequent Falls

Over the years, I've noticed a pattern in fall behavior. Some individuals are just natural frequent fallers; I guarantee this is the category I will one day find myself in, considering the number of falls I have already had. For recurrent fallers, a wheelchair or a walker tends to be the solution, which is unfortunate because for many people the adage "If you don't use it, you lose it" couldn't be more accurate.

Wheelchairs and walkers can be cumbersome around the home, especially if it is not designed for these types of accommodations, which means that, more than likely, your loved one will try to get up and walk around without their walker because it is just easier than having to try to maneuver throughout the home.

For frequent fallers, accessibility is critical. Recreating the space they live in to ensure mobility and safety is essential. While the home may not be designed to meet the needs that come with mobility issues, there are ten ways you can adapt a space:

1. Increase the amount of seating throughout the home.

2. Declutter spaces and ensure clear pathways.

3. Make sure carpet and rugs are flush to the floor.

4. Install grab bars in the bathroom and railings on both sides of stairs.

5. Install lighting throughout the home so that all spaces are illuminated.

6. Move food and essential everyday items to lower shelves.

7. Use a bedside commode to limit trips to the bathroom in the middle of the night.

8. Move the bedroom area to the first floor.

9. Get the person to exercise daily.

10. Have them wear non-slip slippers or house shoes.

Increased accessibility allows an individual to remain as mobile as possible while maintaining their safety. It may seem easier to make someone sit in a wheelchair than to monitor and assist with their mobility regularly, but physical therapy and continued movement can even make providing activities of daily life (ADLs) easier on you.

Sudden Falls

Sudden falls can indicate a progression in the disease process or a sudden-onset illness. Someone who has always been mobile and had an unexpected fall that wasn't related to a mere accident or trip always alerts me that there may be something else happening medically. Often, the culprit is a UTI; however, in more severe cases, a fall can be a symptom of a radical decline in their health. Taking notes and promptly notifying the doctor of this sudden change is the best way to ensure the health and safety of your loved one.

Urinary Tract Infections

There is nothing pleasant about a UTI. Women are more prone to UTIs than men, and dehydration is a leading cause of UTIs in older adults. Bacteria in the bladder cause UTIs. People with incontinence or who have difficulty getting up and going to the bathroom on their own are more at risk for UTIs because of the close contact that adult briefs have with their skin. If you have experienced one, then you know they are quite literally a pain and a nuisance. UTIs will have a much more severe effect on an older adult; delusions, sudden mood or personality changes, and other apparent dementia symptoms are actually common results of the infection.

Many UTIs go undiagnosed because of how closely symptoms resemble dementia, which is unfortunate, both for individuals living with dementia and even for those who are not. For instance, a persistent misconception of old age is that everyone will get dementia. This is a belief held even by people in the medical profession. Dementia is not a normal part of aging, and, if your loved one has a sudden onset of dementia symptoms, you should first rule out the possibility of an infection before their doctor gives them a dementia diagnosis, even if this means you have to be persistent with their doctor. A diagnosis of dementia can become a permanent fixture in their medical chart, so, if they are misdiagnosed, they will continue to be treated as if they do have dementia, even if they don't.

The same goes for individuals who already have a dementia diagnosis. A UTI will make their symptoms worse, and your once sweet and quiet mother is now yelling and throwing chairs—it can happen! While dementia symptoms will have momentary flare-ups from time to time, if you notice that your loved one is showing extreme behavior, they may have a UTI, and they should have their urine tested as soon as possible so they can be prescribed the proper antibiotics.

Here are some suggestions for reducing the risk of UTI:

- Get them to drink plenty of fluids (two to four quarts each day)

- Get them to drink cranberry juice or use cranberry tablets

- Try to keep them from caffeine and alcohol because these irritate the bladder

- Set a timer to remind them to use the bathroom

Memory Care or Disease Progression

There could be many reasons why your loved one is now in your care, but, when you are also handling memory care or a fast disease progression, the ability to watch over them on your own becomes challenged. Around-the-clock care needs require the skills of a trained professional, but knowing when it is time to say you need additional help can be tricky.

As your loved one's health progresses, their ability to assist in their own care will decrease, which means that your regular tasks will start to become more cumbersome and time-consuming. For instance, your mom used to be able to go to the bathroom almost entirely on her own and would only require you to stand there to help her on and off the toilet. But more and more, you find that she needs help finding the toilet paper, putting her clothes back on, and even washing her hands.

While these types of changes usually occur over time, many caregivers won't notice them until the added work starts to burn them out. I've heard many people express hope that their loved one can regain function, and, while this does happen, it mostly occurs with individuals who were affected by a sudden-onset illness or a fall. If they are naturally progressing in their cognitive issue or their disease process, they more than likely will not gain this back and, eventually, will require skilled nursing care.

Mindful Caregiving

Most of the caregiver/care recipient relationship is unspoken, and to be able to identify subtle changes in your loved one's demeanor, or to notice new symptoms in their disease progression, will require a focus on the person rather than the care tasks. Incorporating a person-centered approach to care will help you manage your time in a way that supports both of you in the care routine. Certain aspects of care can be deceptive and can leave you unsure if they are progressing in their disease process or if it is just an accident or mishap. When it comes to medication side effects, falls, UTIs, or memory loss, the way we perceive and initially label new signs and symptoms can have a lasting impact on the individual, which is why it is so important to investigate and find the root cause of new behaviors.

Chapter Seven

How to Have a Conversation about Care

Family members make a lot of assumptions about what will happen to a loved one, or even themselves, without having a conversation with all involved. I've spoken with many older adults who have expressed that they will just let their daughter or their son decide when the time comes. Even if they are saying this with the best intention, not knowing what is going to happen is extremely likely to cause friction in the family. This can also create anxiety and guilt for those left to decide. I firmly believe that there is no right or wrong when it comes to someone's decision to become a caregiver or not. There needs to be autonomy in the choice because ultimately the quality of care that the older adult will receive, and therefore their quality of life, is dependent on the caregiver.

Too often, families wait until they are in an emergency situation before making decisions about their long-term care options, caregiving preferences, and end-of-life care. Generally, these types of conversations can seem scary and initially cause anxiety, but fear of the unknown is just part of being human. In my experience, these conversations end up being more loving and sincere than scary. When held in the right environment and under the right circumstances, a conversation about care will empower all those involved to focus on what really matters, and that is ultimately the person's happiness and well-being.

Advanced care planning is typically talked about the most and focuses on factors like power of attorney, power of health care, and care measures an individual would want taken in the event they are no longer capable of making decisions themselves. However, there are usually many years between our retirement and our passing, which means a multistage plan is needed to ensure that the later years are spent in the way we choose. As I've already mentioned, 86 percent of Americans over the age of sixty-five have expressed the desire to age in their home. To do so successfully will take a financial and medical care plan that supports this decision without creating a burden on those around you. It is one thing to want to age in place if you are independently able to do so, but to think that a loved one will step in to assist because you aren't financially able to hire an in-home caregiver means that your plan is dependent on others' willingness or ability to support you.

There are a lot of factors to consider, which means that these conversations can be easily sidetracked by follow-up questions and deliberations. If you are the caregiver and you want to start a conversation with a loved one, it may be easiest to start by considering how you would answer these types of long-term care questions for yourself. It is never too early to start developing a care plan. Having already gone through the steps and answered key questions will better prepare you, when you talk with your loved one, to keep the conversation on track without having to pause for additional research.

Other family members, friends, and even close neighbors should be made aware of your multistage care plan, but they do not all have to be sitting at the table when you make these decisions. Keeping the number of people in the planning session to a minimum will help keep the conversation focused on the task at hand and allow for moments of reflection. Mindful decision-making is not a luxury. It is something we all have within our power to do, but it can be hard to achieve if there are too many people providing their opinions. Family dynamics are necessary to keep in mind, and, while the number of people at the initial planning session should be low, other immediate family members should also be consulted, especially if they are a part of the person's care plan.

Advocating for yourself as well as your loved one during the conversation/planning session is important because, if anything is not said there, it probably won't be said later when you are actively providing the care. "For the family" is a phrase I've heard come up so many times within a resident care plan meeting, and it often means that one person is taking on the bulk of the responsibility because no one else in the family can or will. Making sure everyone is on the same page, or at least understands their role and why certain decisions have been made, is a great way to prevent future conflicts in the determination of care.

Like many things in life, plans change and evolve over time. Making individual decisions now does not mean that they are set in stone. Many of the planning documents are informal and not legally binding. Keeping your preferences up to date and in a place that is easily accessible will ensure that your choices are honored in the event that you need someone else to uphold them for you.

Asking a Loved One to Make a Plan

To know when or how to have care conversations in itself is hard. Your parent or loved one is the head of the family. They've been making independent decisions for their entire adult life, so to start a conversation that speaks to a loss of independence is understandably uncomfortable. The talk will bring up intimate details of the caregiving process, financial plans and budgets, and even diagnosis and disease treatment plans—topics that can be tiptoed around in everyday life due to their delicate nature, but can't be avoided here.

The way you frame your invitation to them is the first step in having a smooth and productive dialogue. No matter how good your rapport is, this is a serious discussion. While jokes about "old age" may be funny icebreakers, they could also make light of actual circumstances your loved one is facing, and, if approached through humor, you may not get a direct or honest answer. If you show that you genuinely want to listen to them and take their wishes to heart, you've provided them with a safe space to broach topics that they may have been too scared or anxious to bring up themselves.

The focus may be on their care preferences, but the conversation is not just for them. They should be reminded that the discussion will help all involved to be on the same page and prepared to provide care with dignity, and with the understanding that you will be providing care for them in the way that they discussed with you.

_____

_____

_____

_____

Here are a few examples of conversation starters.

[Name] I've been planning for retirement and realized I don't know much about your long-term plans. If I ever have to assist you in making plans or decisions, I want to make sure I'm honoring your wishes. Will you have a care conversation with me?

[Name], your recent diagnosis has made me think a lot about how we can best support you through this new phase of your life. I want to make sure you maintain your independence and make choices based on your preferences when it comes to your care. Will you have a care conversation with me?

[Name], I worry sometimes that I live too far away if something were to ever happen to you. I want to be sure that you have the right resources available to you if you should ever need them. Will you have a care conversation with me?

_____

_____

_____

_____

_____

_____

_____

Designing a Plan

A good place to start when considering a plan is to identify what independence looks like for your loved one. A values list is an excellent way to engage in this conversation. We live in an active and independent society. We are engaged as long as we initiate and are independent as long as we can actively participate. And it isn't until we are no longer able to go to the grocery store or drive over to a friend's house that we may even realize how vulnerable we all really can be. Understanding what independence looks like on an individual level helps prioritize important aspects of the day-to-day routine and highlights areas that would benefit from more focus and planning.

A plan serves as a way to preserve your independence and maintain control in the decisions that will need to be made as you get older. For instance, a big question that gets talked about a lot in the field is the "driving" question. When should a person no longer drive? And should someone else have the right to take the car keys away if they feel the person is unable to operate safely on their own?

Having the ability to drive means they retain their ability to stay active in the community. They can go to the grocery store when they need to or go to the doctor on their own. To take that away without having a conversation beforehand, or without a plan, is a considerable loss and signifies more of a decline in self-sufficiency than necessary. Addressing this question during the planning session and identifying a new way to maintain your loved one's ability to stay active in the community could be all it takes for them to decide for themselves that it is time to stop driving. Understandably, access to public transportation can often be difficult, so ensuring that a close friend or family member can step in to provide rides, or budgeting for a taxi, Uber, or Lyft are two ways to plan. Having this as a reliable second option reassures everyone that they will still able to get out and about if they need to, without risking their safety in the process.

The five main topics that should be planned for are:

1. Housing preference

2. Available finances

3. Socializing

4. Transportation

5. Care preferences

An all-inclusive plan ensures that every aspect of your loved one's life and preferences is acknowledged. Each plan will be unique to the individual's circumstances, so the time to start and the measures that need to be planned will vary.

Housing Preferences

One of the most critical aspects of a care conversation is the housing preference of your loved one. I don't think that this topic is expanded on as much as it needs to be because so many people want to stay in their homes. However, many factors go into living in and maintaining a home as we age. Without the proper measures in place, staying in the house can increase the risk of isolation for that person.

Limiting housing options to the family home also increases the likelihood that family members and close friends will be taking on the bulk of the home upkeep responsibility. Your loved one does not want to be a burden on anyone, and, when they decide they want to stay in the home, more than likely it is through the lens of their current abilities and range of independence. However, without a discussion of who will take on these responsibilities in the event that they are no longer able to do so, it will fall on the primary caregiver to maintain the home, either physically or financially.

For example, if the only thing they told you was that they want to stay in their home, you are then compelled to continue to keep their house for them or pay someone else to do it, out of fear that any other solution will be against their wishes.

To consider that their ability to maintain the home and maneuver safely within it could change over time creates an opportunity to address and find solutions for these types of scenarios together. Discussing your loved one's values about the home setting offers criteria you can use in a later search for alternate long-term care options without the guilt or burden of having to decide for them.

The perception of senior living is too often limited to a nursing home, which in turn narrows the discussion for many, if they believe that the only two choices they have are to stay in their home or move to a nursing home. The next chapter will go over the growing number of housing options available to older adults and identify the characteristics of each. Understanding all the options available to you broadens the possibilities for both care and support later, if your loved one requires it. It also allows for your loved one's values to be more clearly outlined during the conversation. They won't feel they must advocate for themselves to stay in their home because moving to a nursing home isn't an acceptable option for them.

Available Finances

After retirement, many individuals will live on a fixed income, and this income, along with their savings, becomes the funds available to them through every later phase. Budgeting becomes a key aspect of the care conversation and should include flexibility, as certain finances may change over the years. A power of attorney should be identified during the care conversation.

What is a Durable Power of Attorney?

This is a written document, signed by a person, that gives another the legal right to act in conducting the signer's business, including signing papers, checks, title documents, and contracts, handling bank accounts, and other activities in the name of the person granting power.

A power of attorney should be given to someone you trust. A big misconception about the power of attorney is that has to be the same person who oversees the health care decisions—it does not. You can designate two different people for your health care directives and your power of attorney; this is good, since sometimes the person you trust most to make medical decisions for you is the last person you want handling your finances! Another critical point to note is that a power of attorney can be changed at any time the person granting the power chooses, and they can independently make that decision. Relationships change, and to ensure your records appropriately acknowledge this change, you should revisit plans often to ensure that the plan is current and up to date at all times. If you are designating someone as your power of attorney, it is essential that they agree to the terms you have laid out, and fully understand your wishes before accepting the role.

Socialization

So much of our lives involves being with or being around other people. Almost all of us will engage with others daily, whether it is with our families, our friends, or our community. Socializing becomes almost second nature, and often we don't have to think about it or plan for it; we are just able. But what happens when it's no longer as simple as just hopping in the car and going? When once-simple tasks become obstacles? It may not be until your body begins to change that you even notice how many steps you have to go up or down to get out your front door, or how cumbersome and tiring going to the grocery store and carrying all those bags can be.

Older adults living alone at home are at risk of social isolation. Incorporating ideas to maintain social opportunities is important during the planning session. Socializing as a primary need for seniors is not a new concept. Long-term care facilities have incorporated social well-being in residents' care for years. And for good reason! Isolation has several known negative impacts on both health and cognitive functions, and even increases the risk of mortality.

If your loved one wants to remain in their home, staying active in the community and joining clubs or social groups are two great ways to prevent isolation after retirement. For instance, if your mom is in a bridge club or a book club that she attends at a coffee shop or another person's house, is it possible for them to come to pick her up on these days, or could she host the club so that she isn't the one having to leave? To assume that socialization will occur naturally for older adults will leave you responsible for finding ways to keep them active. Include their close friends in the planning session to see how they are willing to intervene to ensure that your loved one can stay active, too. Activities and socializing enhance quality of life and need to be given consideration during the care conversation.

Transportation

An older adult suffers a sense of personal loss when they can no longer continue to drive. Culturally, owning and driving a car symbolizes freedom and independence, which are both important and identifying values held by an individual. The ability to have a car and to get around without assistance promotes a higher quality of life and a continued sense of purpose and self-worth within their community. The fear of losing their independence is so deep that many older adults will knowingly risk their own safety for mobility, and it has been estimated that the annual fatalities of elderly drivers will double in the coming years.[25] The ability to go to doctor's appointments, meet friends for lunch, and go shopping are all important considerations if your loved one has decided to age in place.

To be thoughtful in your conversation and word choices is a good way to approach this delicate topic with your loved one. Framing the situation as being about maintaining their independence should put them at ease and make them less defensive because they won't think you are trying to take something away from them. Before you start the conversation, research and identify safe and reliable transportation options in your loved one's area. Access to transportation is a hot topic among community developers now as it relates to seniors, which means that more and more public programs are becoming available to address the transportation needs of older populations. Here are gentle ways to broach the topic with your loved ones.

> [Your loved one], I know how much you worry about driving to the store every Thursday, so I did a bit of research and found there is a car service that can pick you up from home and drop you back off when you are done. Why don't we give them a call to see if this could work for you?

> [Your loved one], I noticed you have canceled a few appointments recently. If you want to schedule your appointments at [a time convenient for you], we can carpool together because I have [activity] in that part of town at the same time.

> [Your loved one], you haven't used your car in a while, and you will need to do some maintenance to ensure it stays in good condition. Have you considered selling your car?

---

25   Katherine Freund, "Independent Transportation Network: Alternative Transportation for the Elderly," *TR News* 206 (2000): 3–12; Joseph Coughlin and Lisa D'Ambrosio, ed., *Aging America and Transportation: Personal Choices and Public Policy* (New York: Springer, 2012).

The money you receive from the sale could be used to pay for [local transportation program].

_____

_____

_____

_____

_____

_____

_____

_____

_____

_____

_____

_____

_____

_____

_____

_____

Care Preferences

The level of care your loved one needs may change over time or relatively quickly, and because of these types of uncertainties, it is good to know what kind of care preferences your loved one has while they are still able to decide for themselves. Care options are growing to suit the preferences of the large population of Baby Boomers who are requiring skilled care. This expansion of care options opens up a wide variety of opportunities for older adults to age, and receive care, in a place of their choosing.

Starting a conversation on care preferences will depend on multiple factors, and the discussion will look different for everyone. Some of the most important topics to keep in mind include: What type of setting would they prefer? What level of care do they need? What is within their budgetary means? Knowing the answers to these questions will help you narrow your research when it comes time to look into the care options available to your loved one in their community.

A Hundred Questions to Consider during Your Care Conversation

Knowing what to ask during your conversation isn't always easy, so here is a guide to help you ask the right questions with your loved one! This list is to guide your discussion and could be overwhelming if done all in one sitting. Take breaks as you need them, and know that it is okay to come back to the questions at various times. Writing their answers down as they are given will ensure that you can refer to all parts of their plan and preferences later, when you need to. It also helps you explain your loved one's plan to other friends and family who were not in the planning session but will need to know this information.

Housing Questions

- Do you want to live near family?
    - Will this require you to move?
    - Do all of your family members understand your wishes?
    - Have you considered long-term care or in-home care options?
- Is your home adaptable so that you can safely age in place?
    - Is it more feasible to bring the bedroom to the first floor or to install a stair lift?
    - Do you have a walk-in shower?
    - Are there grab bars in the bathroom by the toilet and by the shower?
    - Is there a full bathroom on the first floor?
- What are the normal household chores?
    - Are you able to do the yard work?
    - Are you able to go grocery shopping?
    - Are you able to clean the home?
    - Are you able to cook for yourself?
- Is the home in good condition?
    - Will it need a new roof in a few years?

- Will it need a furnace repair?

- Are the appliances up to date?

- Are the plumbing and electricity functioning properly?

- What are the available resources near your home?

  - What is the closest hospital?

  - Do you have an in-case-of-emergency list?

  - Do you have neighbors you can call on if something happens?

  - What is the closest pharmacy?

Managing Finances

- Do you have a fixed-income plan?

  - Have you established a budget?

  - How many years' worth of savings do you have available?

  - What happens if you run out of money?

  - What bills do you have?

- Do you have a financial advisor?

  - Whom have you granted power of attorney to?

  - Do you have a will or estate plan?

  - Are your beneficiaries up to date?

  - Will you need to pay for in-home care, and how much will it cost?

- Are your financial documents accessible?

- Where can I find your documents if you need them?

- What accounts do you have and where?

- Where are your tax files?

- Do you have a safe deposit box, and where can we find the key?

Socialization

- What is your normal routine?

  - What time do you like to get up in the morning?

  - Do you eat three meals a day?

  - Do you prefer a shower or a bath?

  - Do you like to go out shopping, or have lunch with your friends?

- What aspects of your normal routine could be compromised in the future?

  - Are you able to get in and out of bed on your own?

  - Are you able to climb the steps to the second floor?

  - Will you remember to cook for yourself?

  - Can you still care for your pet?

- What options are available if you are no longer able to independently pursue your routine?

  - Could you hire an in-home aide to assist with light housekeeping and meal prep?

  - Is public transportation an accessible option to get out and about?

- Are close friends or neighbors able and willing to assist?

- Could an Independent Living or Assisted Living community be an option?

Transportation

- What is your driving routine?

  - When and where are your doctor's appointments?

  - How often do you go out shopping?

  - What is the most important thing you need your car for?

- What is your car maintenance routine?

  - Do you have a regular mechanic?

  - Has your vehicle been inspected?

  - Do you keep up with your oil changes?

  - How many miles do you have on the vehicle?

- Where do you keep your vehicle documents?

  - What car insurance do you have?

  - Whose name is on the title?

  - Do you keep your registration in your vehicle?

- What other driving options do you have available?

  - Do you have a car service in your community?

  - Do you have easy access to public transportation?

- Do friends or family live close by who could pick you up?

Care Conversation

- What doctors do you currently see?

  - Do you have a geriatric care manager?

  - Do you have physical therapy?

  - Do you have a list of all your doctors and their contact information?

  - Do you keep track of all your appointments?

- How do you manage your medication?

  - Do you remember to take all your medications?

  - Do you know the name and purpose of each of your medications?

  - What are the side effects of each medication?

  - Where do you get your prescriptions filled?

- Do you have an advance care plan?

  - Do you want to be resuscitated?

  - Are you an organ donor?

  - What are your wishes regarding life-support measures?

  - Do you know who you would want to make health care decisions on your behalf?

- What is your health insurance plan?

- ○ Do you have in-home care or long-term care insurance?

- ○ What services does it cover?

- ○ Does it cover the cost of durable medical equipment?

- ○ Is in-home care covered by your health insurance?

- What long-term care (LTC) options do you prefer?

  - ○ What nursing home or assisted living options are available in your area?

  - ○ Do you want to consider in-home care before a move into an LTC community?

  - ○ What do you want in an LTC community?

    - Private room

    - Pets are welcome

    - Outdoor spaces

    - Activities on site

    - Dining room or restaurant options

    - Memory care

    - Continuing care retirement community

Asking the right questions and developing a plan before a definite need arises will ensure that the decisions you make regarding the direction of your loved one's care are based on their preference and wishes. These types of conversations make us face life transitions that we often try to avoid due to how uncomfortable the topic can make us, but to have them will allow you to focus on what is important when the time comes, which is family.

Additional Resources

The Institute for Healthcare Improvement started the Conversation Project in 2007. Their free, printable starter kits are designed to guide us through a series of questions so that we stay focused on the critical decisions of the end-of-life discussion and so that we open up to an opportunity to spend some time thinking about our values regarding the kind of care we receive.[26]

Honor the Plan

To take the time now to speak with your loved one regarding these aspects of life provides the foundation for a mutually beneficial care plan as your loved one gets older. To create a plan that honors their wishes will help ease your mind as you begin to have to make difficult decisions regarding their care. Relying on the fact that these decisions were thought through and discussed with you allows you to focus on being with your loved one when they need you the most, rather than worrying about whether you are making the right decisions in the direction of their care.

Even if your loved one did not designate you as their power of attorney or their health care advocate, that does not mean they don't trust you. They have their reasons for making this type of

---

26   Institute for Healthcare Improvement, last modified 2019. http://www.ihi.org/.

designation, and their wishes should be respected even if you may not always agree.

Your loved one should look at their plan at least once or twice a year to make sure nothing has changed in their life that would require updating it. You could make sure they are doing this by checking in on some of the questions you think are pertinent to their safety and well-being, or when you start to see changes in their health or functioning. Plus, revisiting the plan will ensure you know exactly what to do in the event you or another member of your family needs to step in as the decision-maker for your loved one.

Chapter Eight

Available Senior Living Options

Throughout our adult lives, we are told to prepare for retirement and to have a life insurance plan for when we die, but what about all the years in between? Why aren't we encouraged more to plan or even think about long-term care supports? We are living in an aging society where life expectancy has significantly increased, and we are living healthier and longer lives; the US Department of Health and Human Services reports that 70 percent of adults over the age of sixty-five will need long-term care support in their lives.[27]

Most people don't plan for long-term care because conversations about advance care planning are difficult. No one wants to believe that there could come a time when they are no longer able to take care of themselves. Often the very thought of ending up in a nursing home is what prevents people from making necessary decisions about their long-term care needs. Unfortunately, avoiding the conversation means that someone else will eventually have to shoulder the responsibility of making these crucial decisions for you.

Aging in place has become the default answer for almost anyone when they are asked about later-life housing plans. This answer is too often based solely on the idea that they don't want to end

---

27 "How Much Care will You Need?" US Department of Health & Human Services, last modified, October 10, 2017. https://longtermcare.acl.gov/the-basics/how-much-care-will-you-need.html.

up in a nursing home. Naturally, I think we all would love to enjoy the comforts of home until the very end, and for some this does happen. However, to make aging in place a sustainable option for you and for your loved one now will take a lot of planning and a lot of money. Nursing homes have become synonymous with long-term care, but, over the past ten years, the senior living industry has seen an influx of care options that break from the traditional nursing-home model that we have come to know.

As family caregivers, you are on the front lines and will take on much of the decision-making power as the care needs of your loved ones begin to increase. The aging process will be different for everyone, and the timing and means with which you have to make decisions will vary. However, there is a progression, and, over the years, your loved one's care needs will become more demanding and complex. The support that a nursing home or memory care unit can provide family caregivers is grossly underrated and even underappreciated. Yes, their reputations are less than ideal, but through research and understanding, family caregivers can become active participants in the care provided to their loved one in these types of settings. The most efficient way to start the research process is with a general idea of what services your loved one needs, a list of their wishes in senior living options, and an estimated budget, which will help you hone in on a home that everyone is sure to be happy with.

Tips on How to Start Your Research

There is a lot of useful information on the internet for individuals ready to begin their senior living research, but that doesn't mean the search will be as easy or straightforward as you would like it to be. With so many options to consider, a simple search can lead you down a rabbit hole of information that will leave you with more questions than answers.

There are four key criteria that you should outline before you start your research.

1. A budget

2. Actual services needed

3. Preferred location

4. List of wishes

Create a Budget

While it is impossible to predict how long you will live, or how great your care needs will be as you get older, you should consider these factors in your budgetary plan. Too many people underestimate the cost of senior living, and I've been in numerous care plan meetings with family members who don't know what to do now that their loved one has run out of money.

1. Count All Assets

As your loved one creates a budget for their retirement needs, consider the amount they have in assets. Many people use the money they receive from the sale of their home and other larger assets to pay for senior living.

Tip: While the sale of the home offers the necessary finances all up front, renting out the home could be a more financially savvy way to stretch their money.

2. Know the Monthly Costs

Living on a fixed income means that every cost needs to be calculated. Uncertainty in the fluctuation of your loved one's health care costs should be considered when making a monthly budget so that funds are secured as needed. Fortunately, many monthly expenses like food, water, and other utility bills will be included in senior living monthly costs.

3. Know What Programs Are Available to Help

Long-term care insurance assists with much of the health care costs associated with senior living, but there are also public programs available to help. Your local Area Agency on Aging, or even State Department of Aging, are both reliable sources and will be able to give you an overview of the programs available in your area.

Assess Needs

The types of care services senior living provides vary across the spectrum of needs, which is great because it means that there is an option for everyone. It is essential to be realistic when identifying the type of care your loved one needs before moving them into a care home. For instance, you may want your loved one to move into assisted living because you are still concerned by the idea of moving them into a nursing home, but the level of care they need is skilled. Another example could be that your loved one only needs the standard of care provided in assisted living, but requires memory care, too. To move them into an assisted living unit that doesn't offer memory care support will affect their quality of life while there because they won't have the type of help they need from staff.

If you are unsure of the level of care your loved one needs, talk to their doctor or consult an occupational therapist who will be able to assess their needs for you and offer recommendations on the types of care that will benefit them the most.

Preferred Location

Identifying the location your loved one will prefer to live in before starting your search will help you narrow the choices. Do they want to stay in the same community where they currently reside? Or are they hoping to move closer to the family? Also consider that senior living prices vary based on location. The question of whether your loved one is willing to move to the next town over for a more affordable living arrangement should be discussed before your search begins.

List of Wishes

Creating a list of criteria or wishes that your loved one wants in their new home is important and ensures that their preferences are honored during the search process. The items on the list should include things like available on-site services, food preferences, location, room type (private or semi-private), pet policies, social engagement opportunities, and a recently built or recently renovated building.

Know Your Options

Independent Living or Fifty-Five and Over Communities

An independent living community offers the freedom to age in place while ensuring access to resources as the need arises. It is a popular option for older adults who are willing and able to move and want the assurance that all their needs will be met as they arise. Each community will look different, and housing styles can range from apartment or condo living to single-family homes or cottages.

These communities will typically have a nurse on site or a health center, access to transportation, and community engagement or recreational pursuits for residents. Residents have the freedom to be as active or non-active as they'd like and can reach out to the community concierge when they need to reserve transportation to a doctor's appointment. Care provision is limited in independent communities. However, mobility and connections to care are accessible.

Assisted Living

An assisted living facility offers the next level of care for individuals who may begin to need additional support in their care routine. Assisted living facilities typically offer units or apartments within the same building, and staff support is on hand to help with medication management, meal preparation, housekeeping, general care assistance, and laundry. Residents have access to three meals a day, daily activities, and around-the-clock health care providers on site.

Assisted living is a good option for individuals who do not require skilled care but do need additional assistance with their care routine. Many residents move into an assisted living facility when in-home care or care from a loved one is no longer as easily managed as it was before.

Nursing Home or Skilled Nursing Centers

The traditional nursing home refers to a skilled nursing facility (SNF). An SNF is designed for individuals who need around-the-clock assistance with their activities of daily living. A resident of an SNF will have 24/7 care support, will have a private or semi-private room (depending on the facility), and will be provided with three meals a day, social engagement pursuits, and on-site nursing support. SNFs are highly regulated and are surveyed by the state they operate in every year to ensure compliance with national and state standards of care.

As care needs progress, nursing facilities offer the kind of care that many family caregivers are no longer able to provide. It is not always clear how to start the search for an SNF, and many people prioritize the quality of the facility before any other consideration. Each state has an ombudsman office whose mission is to uphold the quality of care delivered in nursing homes within its district.[28] To find out who your local ombudsman is, go to ltcombudsman.org.

Memory Care

Memory care units are designed specifically for individuals living with Alzheimer's disease, dementia, and other types of memory problems. Memory care is specialized skilled nursing care that offers 24/7 supervision on a locked unit. Memory care can range between assisted living and skilled nursing, and residents will almost always have a private room, three meals a day, activity engagements, and around-the-clock access to care.

Memory care is a good option for individuals whose memory loss has started to affect other areas of their health and care routine, those who wander, or those who have demonstrated elopement behavior, such as driving the car by themselves without realizing it, or leaving the house without notifying anyone. It is important to note that not all senior living facilities will offer memory care, so be sure to ask during your screening phone call to the facility.

---

28 The National Long Term Care Ombudsman Resource Center, last modified 2019. https://ltcombudsman.org/.

Continuing Care Retirement Community

Continuing care retirement communities (CCRCs) offer an age-in-place model that is adaptable to the changing needs of older adults. They are equipped with independent living, assisted living, skilled nursing, and even memory care units; individuals can move in while still able to independently care for themselves and are guaranteed a place to live and professional care supports to assist them as their needs and abilities change. While this model does tend to be a more expensive care option, there are pricing models, and many individuals use the money they receive from the sale of their home to cover the entrance fee.

A CCRC is an excellent option for individuals who are still active in their communities but want to downsize and not worry about the upkeep of a home. CCRCs tend to be bustling places to live, and many social engagement options seek to cater to all kinds of people. In my experience, they are also situated on beautiful plots of land, which makes you feel like you live at a resort.

Green House Homes

The Green House project was a concept developed by geriatrician Dr. Bill Thomas in 2001. It was designed to put the home back into senior care and has since redefined the way we think about where we live as we age. Their vision is for homes in every community where elders and others enjoy excellent quality of life and quality of care; where they, their families, and the staff engage in meaningful relationships built on equality, empowerment, and mutual respect; where people want to live and work; and where all are protected, sustained, and nurtured without regard to the ability to pay.[29]

Instead of hundreds of residents to a facility, this model maintains homes with no more than ten residents. The small roster ensures that the staff in the home can provide a high quality of life and care to all members of the household. The Green House project is currently only based in the United States and continues to expand into new communities. To learn more about the project, and to find out if there is a home in your community, visit their website at www.thegreenhouseproject.org.

Village Model

The Village model is a model of senior living that promotes healthy aging in place by connecting Village community members with the resources and tools they need to age healthily and happily in their community. It is an empowering model that is led by the members of each Village, and volunteers and staff work to ensure members are connected with the necessary resources they have identified as a community that they need to successfully age in place. The Village map found on their website shows all the currently available Villages, so that you can easily find out if there is one in your loved one's area.[30]

Each Village is run by volunteers and paid staff who work to coordinate access to affordable services for its members. The members decide on the needs of the community, and the model creates a one-stop-shopping experience to ensure members have all they need to age safely and successfully in their own homes.

---

29 The Green House Project, last modified 2019. https://www.thegreenhouseproject.org.

30 Village to Village Network, last modified 2019. https://www.vtvnetwork.org/.

The Villages coordinate via a national organization, Village to Village Network. Learn more from their website at www.vtvnetwork.org.

Shared Housing

The shared housing concept is relatively simple, as homeowners choose to rent out empty rooms in their homes to other older adults who are in need of affordable housing. While made popular by the TV show *The Golden Girls*, shared housing is growing in popularity for both its financial benefits and the built-in companionship that it offers to older adults.

The National Shared Housing Resource Center is a good place to start if your loved one is interested in renting out a room in their home.[31] It is not always easy to know how to go about getting a renter in the home, and especially to find individuals in the same age category as your loved one. The Resource Center has a list of programs in all fifty states that work to connect seniors so that the shared home experience is available for everyone. Find options near you here: nationalsharedhousing.org.

Options Open Opportunities

Nursing homes offer a much-needed service to older adults who require skilled around-the-clock care, but they are not the only senior living option available. Due to an increase in demand to age in place, senior living has adapted its model to suit the

---

31 The National Shared Housing Resource Center, last modified 2019. https://nationalsharedhousing.org/.

changing market trends. The Baby Boomers already have had an impact on the number of options for long-term care. To know what options are available to you and your loved one in your community will allow you to receive support long before around-the-clock care is needed. This added support will ensure both of you can sustain the care arrangement you've agreed upon without burning out or impacting the quality of care you can provide.

Chapter Nine

What to Look for in a Nursing Home

Phew! You've made the decision—or, at the very least, you recognize the potential of a care home to improve quality of life for you and your loved one. Searching for a care home does not mean that your caregiving days are behind you, but it does mean that you will now have the support and expertise your loved one needs so that you can focus on their emotional well-being and, more importantly, your relationship with them.

The search for a good care home can take time, and, while there are companies out there to assist you in making the decision, it is one you can make on your own.

Chapter Eight outlined the different levels of care that can be provided. Here, I will primarily focus on things to look for in your search for a nursing home. It is important that, even if you are searching for an independent or assisted living home, you should still take a tour of their skilled nursing unit if it is also located on site.

Nursing homes in your community will most likely have an online presence, so scoping out what is available through a web search is an excellent place to start. Affordability, availability of services, aesthetics, and reputation are four main criteria to focus on in your research. Including your loved one in the search is important as well. In your conversation with them, they identified their values of what they want in a home, so if that means they want to be able to bring their beloved dog with them, you can weed out all the properties that don't allow pets pretty quickly.

Once you've done your research and have narrowed your list to three to five possible places, it is time to start setting up appointments. I am of two minds. I have heard some professionals recommend just showing up to a property without giving any notice beforehand. Arriving without warning, you are more likely to get a feel for a typical "day-to-day" experience. While this may be true, I think an unscheduled visit is better done after an already scheduled tour has taken place, and you want to revisit the property because you genuinely feel like it would be a good fit for your loved one. Scheduling an appointment guarantees that you will have someone available to show you around and to answer all of your questions.

Having these types of in-depth conversations with your loved one will help you both feel confident and secure in the decision-making process. But let's be honest, making a decision is sometimes much more comfortable than following through with an actual move into long-term care. After all, you have been fully committed to this process for a while now, and in many ways, the experience has redefined your relationship with them. Heavy emotions such as feelings of guilt are healthy, and, I think, stem from the sense of loss or the perception of giving up a part of such an intimate relationship—no matter how difficult the process was, the bonds formed aren't easily broken. Nor should they be; while these feelings are reasonable, there are new ways for you to remain ever present in their care.

Scheduling a Visit

You should always take a tour of the prospective home with your loved one. During your visit, it is normal to see residents walking and wheeling around, nurses at med carts, and you will probably even hear a few call bells or chair alarms going off. Nursing homes are active, and, throughout any given day, family, visitors, staff, and residents are roaming around the halls.

Pay attention to the demeanor of the staff. How are they interacting with the residents? Are they loudly talking to each other in the halls, or are they at their workstations? Does someone welcome you when you walk in, and are they helpful and courteous throughout your visit? The way staff behave and interact with you and with the residents is extremely telling of the culture. If nursing home staff are unhappy with the way things are running, they don't hide it. They might not tell you outright, but, in this instance, actions do speak louder than words.

On your visit, try to sit in during a meal and during an activity. At the activity, are residents engaged? Don't be alarmed if one or two are asleep, as long as the activity staff person is working to engage the others. Also, are staff coming in to take residents to the bathroom? Did they ask them before they took them? Residents may be on a schedule, but they still have the right to choose. All residents should be given the option to be removed from an activity and should be asked if they can be moved before a caregiver touches their wheelchair.

Additionally, is there variety in the calendar? An activities calendar should offer: mental (trivia, reading), emotional (reminiscing, music), physical (exercise), spiritual (church, religious pursuits), and social (spending time with others their age, friends, and family members) activities.

In the dining room, there will be residents who are able to feed themselves and others who require assistance with their feeding. Staff should be engaged with the residents and not focused on holding conversations with other staff members in the room.

Here are a few additional things to look out for while you are there:

- Are their meals on trays? Or do they have a proper place setting?

- Are residents asked what they want to eat before they are served?

- Does the food look hot?

- What do the other residents think of the food?

- Are residents offered clothing protectors? And are they referred to as such, or are staff members calling them "bibs?"

- Are residents who are being assisted in their feeding being told what is on their plate?

Mealtimes are an important part of the culture in a care home, and the way staff interact with the residents can be the most telling while everyone is sitting around the tables. The language staff uses is particularly important for you to listen for. For instance, referring to clothing protectors as "bibs" is frowned upon in the field for its infantile associations.

Questions to Ask on Your Tour:

1. How many residents does each caregiver care for during a shift?

2. How many people live in one room? Do you offer private/semi-private rooms?

3. How much time does the caregiver spend on each resident?

4. What kinds of services do you offer?

5. Can I read your latest survey report?

6. What happens if my loved one runs out of money?

7. What kinds of food do you serve?

8. What kinds of activities do you offer?

9. Am I able to attend care plan meetings?

10. Can I speak with a few of your residents?

11. What is the closest hospital?

12. Do you have a physician on site?

13. Are residents able to choose their own schedules?

Every facility must display its latest survey report in a common area for staff, residents, and visitors to access. If you do not see the report out during your tour, you can always ask the person at the front desk if you can review it. The survey report will notify you of both the strengths and the weaknesses of the facility, recommendations for improvements, and ratings of the facility compared to other homes in the area.

Take Detailed Notes

You will be visiting a variety of nursing homes, so taking detailed notes on your visit will be helpful to you later when you sit and weigh out each option. If they can't go with you on the tour, take your loved one's values list with you. If they can go with you, make sure to write down how they were feeling throughout the tour. Write down your first impressions, and make notes on the sights, sounds, and smells you experienced while walking through the unit.

Making a Decision

You may be the person who is organizing, researching, and navigating the process for your loved one, but it is they who will be moving, so you do want to make sure that they remain in control of the decision and feel confident and comfortable with the choice.

Choosing what nursing home you are going to move into is emotional. Not only is it a significant change, but it is where your loved one will live out the rest of their days. Most likely this factor is weighing on their mind, and their emotions may fluctuate a lot as they move through this process. Their behavior may change, and it is at this time that you will most likely have to lean heavily on the planning conversation you had with them earlier.

An overwhelming process can be handled in a variety of ways by your loved one, and you won't know what it will be like until the process has already started. I was on tour with a close family friend whose mother had decided she wanted to move to a local nursing home. Up until they stepped into the place, she was happy and even excited at the prospect of the move. Her mood changed drastically on the tour, and, by the time she got in the car, she was yelling and accusing her daughter of moving her against her will. Her daughter knew that the care home held many of the values that her mother had expressed wanting and had to rely on this to help her ultimately make the decision. Her mother later admitted that she had seen a few people in wheelchairs and gotten scared that she was going to stop walking if she moved into the care home. A few months later, she was the most active resident there and had a whole new group of friends.

Giving them space and understanding that this is a major transition point in their life is essential. Have as many conversations as they need to have and visit the care home as many times as they need to, so that they have enough time to consider their options and decide where they will make their new home.

If your loved one is unable to decide on their own, understandably it can become complicated to make the decision for them, especially if they have expressed never wanting to end up in a nursing home in the first place. But, if you've done your research and are using your best judgment, with their values in mind, then you will no doubt make the right decision for both you and your loved one. In the next section, however, we will discuss how to deal with those feelings of guilt that can often creep up after moving a loved one into a nursing home.

How to Handle Feelings of Guilt

As your loved one grapples with their loss of independence, as their caregiver, you are battling the same fears and concerns. To witness them losing the ability to take themselves to the bathroom or forgetting who you are is understandably tricky and can take an emotional toll on the relationship you had with this person. Since you are providing care at the same time, it can quickly become your primary focus, and the moments that you have with your loved one may lose the quality that they may have once had. Even after a dementia diagnosis, there are still so many more happy and loving memories to be made together. Seeking professional caregiving support opens the opportunity to refocus your energies on making the most of the time you have with your loved one.

You may still feel uneasy about the decision to move them, even after a conversation about care preferences. A move is another reminder of the changes occurring in their lives, and, for some, a move into a nursing home too directly acknowledges their mortality, which can be scary and emotional. But, no matter how much physical time there is left, there is so much more life to live. To move your loved one into a care home could be the best way for you to relinquish the stress of being a full-time caregiver and refocus your attention and efforts on spending time with them and making them feel comfortable and content during this new phase of their lives.

Access to 24/7 care, daily opportunities for social engagements, and three nutritious meals a day are just some of the many benefits that your loved one will receive upon moving into a skilled nursing center. As the professional care staff takes over, there are still many ways for you to engage in their care to ensure that they are safe and happy in their new environment. The transition may take time for you both, but because of the daily care regimen that staff must follow, your loved one will assimilate to their new home in no time.

Moving to a Nursing Home Can Prevent Isolation

One of the most preventable risks to an older adult's health is isolation. Even those who receive in-home care or live with close friends and family do not receive an adequate amount of socializing throughout the day. In-home caregivers go home, and family will often spend less quality time with their loved one because they need a break from their caregiving duties. This is normal and happens quite a bit.

Over the years, I've watched new residents in the care center flourish, as they have more people to interact with that are their age and have activity options beyond just watching TV or going out for a doctor's appointment. A nursing home will have an entire activities department, and every day of the week there will be a wide range of fun things for your loved one to choose from. For example, there are morning exercise and trivia groups, arts and crafts projects in the afternoon, musical entertainment, and even outings to local shops and restaurants.

Varied social interactions are essential and are increasingly hard to obtain for older adults living in their own home. Activity programs are designed to engage residents physically and mentally so that they maintain the highest functioning levels. Activities staff are also probably the most fun people you will ever meet (and I'm not just saying that!). They are never afraid to start singing a song or put on a silly outfit to ensure that a resident has a good time.

In addition to the pure fun of it all, the activities department is just as regulated as the dining or nursing department, which means that each resident will receive an activities assessment upon moving into the unit that asks them what their preferences are and what hobbies they enjoy. Additionally, staff must keep track of all the activities your loved one attends, and if they find that they aren't getting out as much as they should, the director will add one-on-one intervention to the care plan, which means they will receive personalized social engagements throughout the week.

The activities aren't just for the residents either; family members and friends are encouraged to attend all sorts of musical events, shopping trips, or parties with their loved ones. This is a fun way to engage with them and takes the pressure off you to come up with ideas every time you visit. Plus, the activities department is always looking for an extra set of helpful hands, so if you want to get involved and volunteer, you should speak with the activities director to see if it would be a good fit for you.

Let's Eat! Around the Clock Monitoring of Your Loved One's Nutrition

Loss of appetite is common in older adults, particularly for individuals living with dementia or Alzheimer's. For those individuals living at home or with close friends and family, their diet becomes dependent on whatever the caregiver can serve. It is difficult to make food and exercise lifestyle changes if the caregiver doesn't already incorporate healthful habits into their daily routine, so the older adult in their care will often have to assimilate to their lifestyle.

In a care center, a registered dietitian assesses each resident. Dietitians are trained in geriatric needs and understand common dementia symptoms such as loss of appetite. Each resident then is given a specific nutritional diet that assists them in either maintaining their current weight, losing weight, or gaining weight. Each resident is also offered three meals a day and snacks between meals, not to mention anything good that the activities team cooks up that week!

Stay Active in Their Care

While nursing homes may have a less than ideal reputation, they aren't all that bad! I've met so many wonderful and caring direct-care workers over the years who provide the best care for the residents. Still, even as they move their loved ones in, many family members express hesitation about the decision. The attention to your parent's or loved one's needs is of the utmost importance!

The best way to ensure your loved one is receiving the best care is to remain active in the care process.

- Visit as often as you can.

- Attend loved one's care plan meetings whenever possible.

- Check in to make sure that they have enough of their favorite shampoo, snacks, etc., on hand.

- If the center is responsible for laundry, write their name and room number with a laundry marker in each article of their clothing.

- Even if you live too far away to visit frequently, schedule time to video-conference or call your loved one. You can even call in to their care plan meeting and discuss their care with the team if you have any questions or concerns.

- Get to know the staff who are caring for your loved one.

A care plan meeting brings together each department head, the resident, and their family members to discuss progress or changes in the resident's routine. It is scheduled for each resident every quarter and can be attended either in person or by phone, depending on the facility. It is a great forum to get to know the staff taking care of your loved one and gives you an opportunity to express any concerns you may have about the direction of their attention. The facility should notify you of the care conference in advance so that you have time to schedule around it. The meeting happens even if you aren't in attendance, but the conversation is always much more robust if family members are present.

Know Their Rights and Your Local Ombudsman

Senior living is one of the most highly regulated industries, and residents living in SNFs have rights that are both federally- and state-mandated. To know these rights and to advocate for them on behalf of your loved one is an excellent way to stay active in their care.

In 1987, the Nursing Home Reform Law was signed, and declared that each resident living in a long-term care home would receive both quality of care and quality of life.[32] The Nursing Home Reform Law established the following rights for nursing home residents:

- The right to freedom from abuse, mistreatment, and neglect

- The right to freedom from physical restraints

- The right to privacy

- The right to accommodation of medical, physical, psychological, and social needs

- The right to participate in resident and family groups

- The right to be treated with dignity

- The right to exercise self-determination

- The right to communicate freely

- The right to participate in the review of one's care plan, and to be fully informed in advance about any changes in care, treatment, or status in the facility

- The right to voice grievances without discrimination or reprisal

If you believe any of these rights have been violated by staff at the nursing home your loved one resides in, you can advocate on their behalf by reporting the violation to the director of nursing of the facility. If you do not feel comfortable addressing such a

---

32 Martin Klauber and Bernadette Wright, *The 1987 Nursing Home Reform Act* (Washington, DC: AARP Public Policy Institute, 2001). Also see, Helen Meenan, Nicola Rees, and Israel Doron, *Towards Human Rights in Residential Care for Older Persons* (New York: Routledge, 2016).

person or other staff directly, you can call your local ombudsman to report the incident with the option to remain anonymous.

Many nursing homes celebrate Resident Rights Month every October, but reviewing these rights with your loved one often will ensure that they are aware of their rights and can identify if they are being violated. Resident rights activities are some of my favorites, and it is my experience that the residents leave the activity feeling confident and empowered to advocate for themselves and their fellow residents.

Below are just a few questions to get you started:

1. True or **False**—Once a resident enters a nursing home, they lose their rights.

2. Residents' rights in nursing homes in the US are protected at which level? **Federal and State**

3. If a diabetic in a nursing home wants to have a piece of cake against physician's orders, what should the nurse do?

    - **allow them to have it**

    - give them something sugar-free

    - call the doctor for advice

4. **Yes** or No—If a nursing home resident has food left on her face after a meal, is this a violation of her rights?

5. **True** or False—Technically, calling a resident "sweetie" or "honey" is a violation of their rights.

With professional caregivers and around-the-clock care provided to your loved one in a nursing home, it can be difficult to gauge how you can adequately protect and care for them. They still need you, and the quality of life they will have in a nursing home setting directly correlates with the family and friends' willingness to visit and engage once they have moved into the home. There are many ways for you to be active in your loved one's care, support them in their social engagements, and advocate on their behalf by learning and protecting their rights.

Making the Decision Could Help Both You and Them!

Deciding to move a loved one into a care center is not easy to do. Too often, a family caregiver is left to judge without knowing the wishes of their loved one. Holding feelings of uncertainty or even guilt is common. I've watched so many family members experience these emotions, but you don't have to feel alone in the process. This is a regular occurrence, and deciding to seek additional help in the care of your loved one is often the best caregiving decision you can make for them and you. Many older adults in need of care support experience isolation and loss of appetite. Care homes are designed to address such dementia symptoms, and individuals living with dementia will receive a personalized care plan that seeks to address these concerns. No matter the reason for seeking additional support in your caregiving duties, it is important to trust your own decisions.

Chapter Ten

Once a Caregiver, Always a Caregiver

The experience of caregiving leaves us with a new perspective on life as it allows the care provider a glimpse of the vulnerable ways our bodies can change over time and humbles us with the question, who will do this for me one day? An understanding of what it takes to give your time, patience, and energy over so that another person can live a dignified and independent lifestyle is precious. And, while the caregiver takes on many roles, the bond that is created is something that will never break. You will carry this experience with you always, and it will change you in ways that you may never truly understand, but the kindness and compassion I have seen as the result of a loved one living with dementia is universal among family caregivers.

There are many different ways caregivers handle the experience of caregiving once their loved one has passed away. Some people want nothing more to do with the experience. They are tired, and the time they spent providing care may have caused trauma or feelings of fear, anger, or sadness. The loss of their loved one may offer some relief from the process, but they can still be burdened by memories of difficult times spent trying to provide care. While time heals, the memories you have of your experience can easily take over any more familial memories you accrued before becoming their caretaker.

You are not alone in your feelings, and there are others out there who have shared their experience in hope to offer validation that you are not alone. Too many caregivers have expressed regret or shame about the decisions they made while providing care, and while not all behavior is acceptable, those decisions made out of love were made with your loved one's best interest at heart. The fact that you were there for them during the process was enough in itself to be a commendable act of kindness and generosity, and while, yes, for some families, the sentiment of "that is just what you do" is right, for many others it is not. Family dynamics are an essential aspect of the caregiving conversation. If you, the caregiver, are still processing familial relationships that were not loving or were not always reliable on top of having to handle your loved one forgetting who you are, it is very easy to blend the diagnosis with the person, even after they have passed away.

The passing of a loved one you provided care for will bring about a mixture of emotions, and many people will need time to process their experience and become reacquainted with a non-caregiving routine. Because it is such a defining part of your life, I am a firm supporter of the notion that, once you've become a caregiver, you are always a caregiver. And even if you never look back to your caregiving days and you choose to move on from the experience, a part of you has changed. In this last chapter, we will discuss various ways you can use the knowledge you gained as a caregiver to memorialize your experience.

How to Memorialize Your Experience as a Caregiver

To suddenly stop providing care, or even thinking about it, will take some getting used to. While you grieve the loss of a loved one, you are left with a mixture of feelings as the time and energy that you put into this season of your loved one's life has come to an end. There are a lot of emotions to grapple with and, while grief hurts, to move through the process is healthy and offers you the chance to reflect on the time you spent together. The extra time you now have will allow you to refocus and reprioritize things in your own life, and while situations may "go back to normal," you may also find that you are looking to take what you learned from the experience and do something with your newfound knowledge and expertise. Your caregiving journey matters, and does not easily come to an end once the person you've cared for passes away. This section will go over a few of the many options available to you as you start your new chapter.

Spend fifteen minutes writing down ten activities/ventures you've wanted to try or start.

1. _____

2. _____

3. _____

4. _____

5. _____

6. _____

7. _____

8. _____

9. _____

10. _____

The Other Things You Love

No matter how long you spent being your loved one's caregiver, there were things in your life that you had to put on hold so you could be present and focused. The experience can be emotional and draining, and now that they have peacefully moved on, you don't ever have to look back on that time again if you don't want to. I've met so many people who expressed being unable to think about it because the experience was so challenging for them, and I think it is important to embrace these feelings if you have them. You did your part and went up and beyond the call of duty, so take this moment to refocus that energy into an aspect of your life that you design for yourself.

You were there for your loved one when they needed you most; this in itself is a job well done. The experience required you to carve time out of your routine to be able to accomplish everything; consider how you want to spend this carved-out time now that you are no longer providing care. Do you want to start a new hobby? Do you want to spend more time with your family? Trust that you deserve to focus on you and take time to explore the potential pathways ahead of you.

Write a Book

Whether you have a way with words or not, writing a book based on your experience as a family caregiver is an empowering way to memorialize this time with your loved one. The moments that you spent providing care are still within you, waiting to be shared. To record these moments and memories offers you a beautiful way to remember and process the experience you went through.

A book on caregiving also becomes a tool and resource for others who are experiencing the caregiving journey and are seeking advice from others who have already gone through the process. If you don't know where to start, check out books by others who have shared their experience, like Carol Bradley Bursack's book *Minding Our Elders* or any of the books in the AlzAuthors catalog.

Write Their Story

Your loved one's dementia diagnosis and health progression is only a fragment of their life story. Many people express not wanting to remember their loved one with Alzheimer's or other forms of dementia this way, and that they would prefer to look back on times pre-diagnosis. A meaningful way to do this is to write their biography. Their life story is worthy of being told, including the parts they may not have been able to remember.

You can start by writing down stories they told or gathering pictures and memorabilia that they kept around their home. Researching and collecting items is a fun way to reengage other family members to get their side of the story. To look back on your loved one's life is a humbling practice and offers a good reminder of how much they lived and loved during their time here.

Become an Advocate

To work so closely with someone living with a form of dementia gives you a unique perspective on what the needs are for these individuals and an understanding of how others generally treat them. To use this knowledge to advocate on behalf of both them and the larger population of individuals living with dementia is a noble cause. The awareness you can bring to this issue is so important, and to share your experience is invaluable.

Dementia is not the only cause you can support. As a family caregiver, you know firsthand the demands caregivers face and can identify where added support is needed. To share your story with businesses and local government and to advocate on behalf of all family caregivers is a way for you to support others who are going through the same effort as you.

Start a Support Group

Support groups offer a safe space to work through and discuss emotions and experiences with others who have gone through similar situations. There can never be too many support groups because there are a million different experiences and topics that can occur during the caregiver's journey. To start a support group of your own creates this space for others who may not know where to turn on any given topic. Offering a place for people to go where they can safely discuss their experience without judgment is a beautiful way to give back.

While many support groups have a broader theme that caters to a particular audience, like "family caregivers of someone living with Alzheimer's" or "Parkinson's Disease," you can choose a topic that is much more targeted; for instance, maybe you struggled with the memory loss aspect of your loved one's diagnosis progression. Organize a support group that discusses just this aspect of the process.

Support a Charitable Cause

There are a variety of foundations and charities that work on dementia. As there are many forms of dementia, each type has its foundational support, like the Alzheimer's Association or the Lewy Body Dementia Foundation. These foundations raise money for research and educational resources for individuals who are diagnosed and for their family members.

There are also different ways you can show your support, for instance, the Alzheimer's Association holds the Walk to End Alzheimer's every year in cities all across the US. Or, if you want to host a fundraiser, many of the organizations will offer assistance to you on their website. For instance, the Parkinson's Foundation provides several options for individuals who want to donate their way, including ideas on how to throw a party, organize a community walk, or host an online fundraising event.

Donate Your Care Items

Do you find yourself surrounded by the care items you needed while providing for your loved one? Adult briefs, Ensure, shower chairs, bedside commodes, grab bars, stair lifts, walkers, and wheelchairs are only a few of the items your loved one may have needed while they were in your care. These items provided much-needed assistance in the provision of care and offered you the support you required to do your job effectively. These items are near universal in the care of older adults, but are expensive, and many people can't afford them.

Donating your loved one's care items is a charitable way to give back to the community, and to put to continued good use the items that assisted you so greatly. If you don't know of a local donation closet that accepts these items you can reach out to your local Agency on Aging, hospital, or senior centers, who may be better connected to sources who will accept your donations.

Make It a Career

The aging field is vast and offers so many different career choices for those who are interested in working with older adults. As a caregiver, your knowledge and experience are resources that the aging field needs if it is to support the growing number of older adults. If you aren't sure where to start, volunteering is a smart way to utilize your skills while you make professional connections in the field. Nursing homes are always in need of volunteers, and your keen eye and understanding of the disease progression make you an excellent candidate to work with the residents.

If you are confident that you want to change your career and are ready to make the switch, hone in on what aspect of the aging field you would want to work in. Depending on the pathway you choose, you may want to consider going back to school for a degree or certificate program. The need is vast, so you are sure to find a position that is right for you.

Thank You

Thank you for being a caregiver. You are needed more than you could ever possibly know. Your loved one is lucky to have you on their side as they navigate this new phase of their life. While others may not always know how to help you, one of the greatest things I hope we can do is to acknowledge your hard work and show you our appreciation. There is no one-size-fits-all description of a family caregiver, and I say this because no matter what type of care you provide, you deserve recognition for the work that you do. You are managing a process that does not have a detailed guidebook and will take you down roads you never thought you would have to travel. You will no doubt see a side of your loved one that you didn't know was there, and together you will learn more about each other.

My hope for you is to look back on your experience fondly and to take away a greater sense of self and understanding of how precious our lives can be. Dementia is a complex diagnosis that brings with it a set of challenges that are often difficult to understand and work through; however, the love and laughter that I have witnessed and experienced with individuals living with dementia is the purest kind of interaction I've ever had. Despite all the frustrations, late nights, and lost memories, your loved one is there with you in the moment. Whether they can say it or not, they are grateful to have you by their side to help them as they struggle with loss of their functions and independence. As their caregiver, you offer them a chance to maintain their dignity throughout the remainder of their life.

Acknowledgments

I started the Upside to Aging website to share and connect with others who have experienced the love and laughter of someone living with dementia. Writing this book was a beautiful and challenging process and honestly a feat I never dreamed of accomplishing. I am so so fortunate to have this opportunity to share my practice with you, and while most of this book offers the sentiment of finding support, I too appreciate the support that was given to me through this process.

To my favorite person, my husband, Kevin A. Wisniewski. He listened to me read off so many of these paragraphs with more patience than I probably deserved. His encouragement and enthusiasm throughout this process (and all the other eight years' worth of projects he's supported me through) is what inspires me to write on. I am thankful every day that he is my partner.

To Rutherford, my Handsome Man (and loving cat). Thank you for sitting next to me as I wrote even when you only wanted to play.

To Mango Publishing, for offering me the chance to share my work with all of you! I am grateful to work with a wonderful team whose mission is to explore new ideas and start conversations with their readers.

To Carol Bradley Bursack, whom I've gotten to know through her work to educate and support family caregivers. I'm so grateful for her support and appreciative that she took the time to share her story with all of you by authoring the foreword of this book.

To Jefe, my mentor and first boss in the field, Sandi Bradford. She offered me a wonderful chance to work in activities while I was still fresh out of high school. Her compassion, empathy, and respect for older adults were foundational in my understanding of dementia, and I will be forever grateful that she was willing to teach me all that she knew.

To the residents and staff at the Methodist Country House. I learned so much from you all, and the years I spent working in the activities department were a wonderful introduction to my career in aging, notably, to Ora who was my first friend there.

To Cohort 8, the faculty, and staff at the Erickson School at UMBC, I learned so much from all of you, and I reflected on so many lessons and conversations we had while writing this book.

To my parents, Donna and Mike LeGrand, whose support has been so encouraging. I don't think my mom has missed sharing a single one of my posts! To Adam, my brother, who thinks writing the book is cool, and tells me so! And to my Grandmom, Sarah Lovenduski, who inspires me every day, and who I look up to the most.

To my fantastic family and friends who checked in and listened as I worked through the writing process. All of your support means the world, and I look forward to sharing this book with you.

References

AlzAuthors. 2019. Accessed 2019. www.alzauthors.com.

Alzheimer's Association. 2019. *Caregiver Stress.* Accessed 2019. https://www.alz.org/help-support/caregiving/caregiver-health/caregiver-stress.

American Association of Retired Persons (AARP). *AARP Livable Communities.* "Baby Boomer Facts on 50 Livable Communities and Aging in Place." AARP. 2018. https://www.aarp.org/livable-communities/info-2014/livable-communities-facts-and-figures.html.2018/.

American Public Health Association, "Fact Sheet: Prescription Medication Use by Older Adults" MedScape, accessed April 1, 2019. https://www.medscape.com/viewarticle/501879.

Bursack, Carol Bradley. Miding Our Elders. 2019. https://mindingourelders.com.

Center for Disease Control. *State of Aging and Health in America 2013.* Division of Population Health, US Department of Health and Human Services, Atlanta: Center for Disease Control, 2013.

Cohn, D'vera, and Jeffrey S. Passel. 2018. "A record 64 million Americans live in multigenerational households." Pew Research Center, 5 April 2018. http://www.pewresearch.org/fact-tank/2018/04/05/a-record-64-million-americans-live-in-multigenerational-households/.

Coughlin, Joseph and Lisa D'Ambrosio, ed. *Aging America and Transportation: Personal Choices and Public Policy.* New York: Springer, 2012.

Dementia Mentors. 2019. Accessed 2019. https://www. dementiamentors.org.

Family Caregiver Alliance. 2019. https://www.caregiver.org.

Feinberg, Lynn, and Rita Choula. "Understanding the Impact of Family Caregiving on Work." *Fact Sheet 271*. Washington, DC: AARP Public Policy Institute, 2012. http://www.aarp. org/content/dam/aarp/research/public_policy_institute/ ltc/2012/understanding-impact-family-caregiving-work-AARP-ppi-ltc.pdf.

Freund, Katherine. "Independent Transportation Network: Alternative Transportation for the Elderly." *TR News* 206 (2000): 3–12.

Gasfriend, Jody. "Survival for the Sandwich Generation: Navigating the hidden costs for working caregivers." *Salon*, 21 May 2018. Accessed 2019. https://www.salon.com/2018/05/20/ surviving-the-sandwich-generation-navigating-hidden-costs-for-the-working-caregiver/.

"How Much Care will You Need?" US Department of Health & Human Services. 10 October 2017. https://longtermcare.acl.gov/ the-basics/how-much-care-will-you-need.html/.

Institute for Healthcare Improvement. "The Conversation Project." *Starter Kits*. 2007. Accessed 2018. https:// theconversationproject.org/starter-kits/.

International Alliance of Carer Organizations (IACO). 2019. Accessed 2019. https://internationalcarers.org.

Klauber, Martin, and Bernadette Wright. *The 1987 Nursing Home Reform Act*. Washington, DC: AARP Public Policy Institute, 2001. Accessed 2019. https://www.aarp.org/home-

garden/livable-communities/info-2001/the_1987_nursing_
home_reform_act.html.

National Alliance for Caregiving and AARP. "Caregiving in
the US 2015." Research, National Alliance for Caregiving
and AARP, 2015. http://www.caregiving.org/wp-content/
uploads/2015/05/2015_caregivingintheUS_Final-Report-
June-4_WEB.pdf.

National Association of Area Agencies of Aging. 2016. Accessed
2019. https://www.n4a.org.

Parker, Kim, and Eileen Patten. *The Sandwich Generation
Rising Financial Burdens for Middle-Aged Americans.*
Washington, DC: Pew Research Center Social and Demographic
Trends, 2013).

Accessed 2019. http://www.pewsocialtrends.org/2013/01/30/
the-sandwich-generation/.

Respect Caregivers Time Coalition (ReACT) and AARP.
*Supporting Working Caregivers: Case Studies of Promising
Practices.* Case Study, Respect Caregivers Time Coalition
(ReACT) and AARP, 2017. https://respectcaregivers.org.

Rossato-Bennett, Michael, dir. *Alive Inside: A Story of Music
and Memory.* Documentary. Projector Media and the Shelley &
Donald Rubin Foundation, 2014. DVD.

SeniorLiving.org. *1900–2000: Changes In Life Expectancy
In The United States.* 2018. Accessed 2019. https://www.
seniorliving.org/history/1900-2000-changes-life-expectancy-
united-states/.

The Green House Project. *Reinventing Care. Empowering Lives.*
2019. Accessed 2019. https://www.thegreenhouseproject.org.

The National Caregiver Alliance and AARP Public Policy Institute. *Caregiver Profile: The Millennial Caregiver.* Washington, DC: The National Caregiver Alliance and AARP Public Policy Institute, The National Caregiver Alliance and AARP Public Policy Institute, 2015.

The National Consumer Voice. 2019. Accessed 2019. https:// theconsumervoice.org.

The National Long Term Care Ombudsman Resource Center. 2019. Accessed 2019. https://ltcombudsman.org/.

The National Shared Housing Resource Center. 2019. Accessed 2019. https://nationalsharedhousing.org.

The Pioneer Network. 2019. Accessed 2019. https://www. pioneernetwork.net.

US Department of Health & Human Services. *Caregiver Resources & Long-Term Care.* 2017. Accessed 2019. https:// www.hhs.gov/aging/long-term-care/index.html.

University of Missouri Extension. *Baby Boomers (born 1946– 1964).* n.d. Accessed 2019. http://extension.missouri.edu/ extcouncil/documents/ecyl/meet-the-generations.pdf.

—. *Silent Generation / Traditionalists (born before 1946).* n.d. Accessed 2019. http://extension.missouri.edu/extcouncil/ documents/ecyl/meet-the-generations.pdf.

Validation Training Institute, Inc. n.d. Accessed 2019. https:// vfvalidation.org.

Village to Village Network. 2019. Accessed 2019. https://www. vtvnetwork.org.

Wisniewski, Molly. The Upside to Aging. 2019. *Caregiving With Dignity*. Accessed 2019. https://theupsidetoaging.com.

About the Author

Molly Wisniewski is a writer and consultant in the aging services. She received her M.A. in the Management of Aging Services at the Erickson School, UMBC. She has over ten years' experience working with seniors in a variety of settings including Continuing Care Retirement Communities, Public Policy, and Consumer Advocacy. She began her career with a mentor dedicated to the teaching of Resident Rights and a strong advocate for the quality of life and care for seniors living in nursing homes. As an activity professional, she was continuously humbled by the joy, kindness, and compassion individuals living with dementia have in their heart and their willingness to share this love with all those they meet. Her mission is to help caregivers cultivate the same type of relationships with the older adults living with Alzheimer's or another form of dementia in their life. Her blog the *Upside to Aging* is dedicated to sharing an alternative and more positive side to aging.

CPSIA information can be obtained
at www.ICGtesting.com
Printed in the USA
BVHW081910160719
553596BV00001B/1/P